The Nervous System

STRUCTURE AND FUNCTION IN DISEASE
MONOGRAPH SERIES

ABNER GOLDEN, M.D.
Series Editor

Available Volumes
Golden & Maher: THE KIDNEY

STRUCTURE AND FUNCTION
IN DISEASE
MONOGRAPH SERIES

The Nervous System

DAVID M. ROBERTSON, M.D.

Professor of Pathology (Neuropathology)
Queen's University
Kingston, Ontario

HENRY B. DINSDALE, M.D.

Associate Professor of Medicine (Neurology)
Chairman, Division of Neurology
Queen's University
Kingston, Ontario

The Williams & Wilkins Company • *Baltimore 1972*

Made in the United States of America

Library of Congress Catalog Card Number 72-88118
S.B.N. 683-07299-4

Composed and printed at
Waverly Press, Inc.
Mt. Royal and Guilford Avenues
Baltimore, Md. 21202 U.S.A.

FOREWORD

The Nervous System by Robertson and Dinsdale is the second member of the *Structure and Function in Disease Monograph Series.* The individual volumes in this series are united by the conviction that an appreciation of the reciprocal relationship between anatomic alteration and disturbance of function is requisite to the understanding of human disease. Each is the combined effort of a pathologist and an internist, selected primarily with regard to their experience in medical education.

The objectives of the series are perhaps best realized by co-authors who have worked together closely and have learned to listen to and to comprehend the points of view of each other's disciplines. Drs. Robertson and Dinsdale fit this bill admirably. They were classmates in medicine at Queen's University, and have served that university for a decade as members of the faculty. For several years, they have shared responsibility for organizing the coordinated teaching program of Clinical Neurosciences in second year medicine at Queen's, and this volume is in many respects an outgrowth of that effort.

David M. Robertson trained in General Pathology at Queen's, in Neurology at Toronto General Hospital, and in Neuropathology at the National Hospital, Queen Square, London, and at Duke University. He is Professor of Pathology at Queen's University, with principal responsibility in Neuropathology. He has recently been appointed Associate Editor of *Laboratory Investigation.*

Henry B. Dinsdale received postgraduate training in Internal Medicine at Queen's, in Neurology and Psychiatry at Maudsley Hospital and the National Hospital, Queen Square, London, and then in Neurology and Neuropathology in the Neurology Unit at Boston City Hospital. He is Associate Professor of Medicine and Chairman of the Division of Neurology in the Department of Medicine at Queen's.

ABNER GOLDEN, M.D.
Series Editor

PREFACE

Neuropathology and the clinical neurosciences have traditionally worked in close harmony, undoubtedly related to the unifying influence of neuroanatomy, the keystone to interpretation of disorders of the nervous system. As the fields of physiology, biochemistry, and, most recently, virology have extended our understanding of neurologic disease, the interdisciplinary interaction has tended to grow in strength and importance.

In this monograph we have attempted to provide the medical student with information and principles essential to a basic understanding of the interplay of etiologic factors, and of the structural and functional alterations that underlie the clinical manifestations of neurologic disease processes. It has been assumed that the student will have previously attained a reasonable understanding of the structure and function of the normal human nervous system. We also believe that the student must have a concurrent opportunity to test what he has read by studying individual patients in a clinical setting and should be guided to explore a few selected disease entities in depth, both clinically and pathologically.

As in other monographs in this series, the limitations of space have dictated a careful selection of those aspects to be discussed. The emphasis has been on areas in which structural and functional correlates are best illustrated, keeping in mind the relative frequency of different entities and those fields in which there has been recent progress in our understanding of basic mechanisms. We recognize that the selection has been to some extent arbitrary and we realize that others might choose different models. We have deliberately avoided the temptation to provide lengthy and detailed descriptions of the morphologic changes, emphasizing instead only those points essential to understanding pathogenesis. Similarly, clinical manifestations are mentioned to illustrate the correlative approach and are not intended in any way to be encyclopedic. Certain controversial subjects have been simplified or discussed from a point of view that might well ultimately be proven incorrect.

We wish to thank Dr. David A. Rosen and Dr. D. G. Wollin for providing the fundus photographs and x-rays, respectively. We are particularly grateful to Mr. Norman Meyers for his capable assistance with the photographic material, and to Mrs. Pat Scilley for typing the manuscript. We wish to acknowledge, too, the support and inspiration of our students and colleagues at Queen's University.

DAVID M. ROBERTSON
HENRY B. DINSDALE

GENERAL REFERENCES

ADAMS, R. A., AND SIDMAN, R. L. Introduction to Neuropathology. Blakiston-McGraw-Hill Book Co., New York, 1968.

BABEL, J., BISCHOFF, A., AND SPOENDLIN, H. Ultrastructure of the Peripheral Nervous System and Sense Organs. Atlas of Normal and Pathological Anatomy. C. V. Mosby Co., St. Louis, 1970.

BLACKWOOD, W., DODDS, T. C., AND SOMMERVILLE, J. C. Atlas of Neuropathology. 2nd edition. E. & S. Livingstone, Ltd., Edinburgh, 1970.

BLACKWOOD, W., McMENEMEY, W. H., MAYER, A., NORMAN, R. M., AND RUSSELL, D. S. Greenfield's Neuropathology. 2nd edition. Edward Arnold, Ltd., London, 1963.

BODIAN, D. Neurons, circuits, and neuroglia. *In* The Neurosciences, a Study Program. Ed. by G. C. Quarton, T. Melnechuk, and F. O. Schmitt. The Rockefeller University Press, New York, 1967.

BRAIN, THE LATE LORD, AND WALTON, J. N. Brain's Diseases of the Nervous System. Oxford University Press, London, 1969.

HAYMAKER, W. Bing's Local Diagnosis in Neurological Diseases. C. V. Mosby Co., St. Louis, 1969,

HOLMES, G. Introduction to Clinical Neurology. E. & S. Livingstone, Ltd., Edinburgh, 1968.

MERRITT, H. H. A Textbook of Neurology. Lea & Febiger, Philadelphia, 1967.

MINCKLER, J. (Ed). Pathology of the Nervous System. McGraw-Hill Book Co., New York, Vol. I, 1968, Vol. II, 1971.

NOBACK, C. R. The Human Nervous System. McGraw-Hill Book Co., New York, 1967.

PEELE, T. L. The Neuroanatomic Basis for Clinical Neurology. 2nd edition. McGraw-Hill Book Co., New York, 1961.

SLAGER, U. T. Basic Neuropathology. The Williams & Wilkins Co., Baltimore, 1970.

SPILLANE, J. D. An Atlas of Clinical Neurology. Oxford University Press, London, 1968.

TEDESCHI, C. G. (Ed). Neuropathology. Methods and Diagnosis. Little, Brown & Co., Boston, 1970.

VINKIN, P. J., AND BRUYN, G. W. Handbook of Clinical Neurology. Vol. I. Disturbances of Nervous Function. North-Holland Publishing Co., Amsterdam, 1969.

CONTENTS

1

AN INTEGRATED APPROACH TO DISORDERS OF THE HUMAN NERVOUS SYSTEM

Although much about its organization remains unknown, the nervous system, more than any other, allows one to interpret disturbed function in terms of specific anatomic structure. Examination of the patient with neurologic disease should be designed to elicit symptoms and signs, and then to interpret them in terms of disordered function which can be related to anatomic regions in the nervous system. However, it must be remembered that the patient's complaints have to be considered not only in terms of the way the patient reacts to structural changes within his body, but also in recognition of the social and environmental factors which play such a large part in human disease. There must be careful elicitation and interpretation of all factors relevant to the patient's problems if investigation and treatment are to proceed in a logical manner.

FACTORS INFLUENCING THE EXPRESSION OF STRUCTURAL DISEASE OF THE NERVOUS SYSTEM

A number of factors determine whether or not structural damage causes neurologic dysfunction. Some regions of the nervous system, such as the frontal lobe, can suffer sizable lesions without producing noticeable symptoms ("silent areas"), whereas equivalent or even smaller lesions located elsewhere, for example, along the course of a cranial nerve, produce an obvious and distressing complaint such as diplopia.

Another important element is the speed of evolution of the lesion. The nervous system may be able to adapt to a large extent to a slowly evolving lesion, whereas the same lesion appearing suddenly results in greater immediate clinical impairment.

The age of the patient is important. Young children recover from central nervous system damage with greater ease and resilience than

1

adults. In some instances, this is because rigid localization of function within the cerebral hemispheres does not develop until the child reaches a certain chronologic age, which may vary between individuals, and presumably represents a stage of maturation and myelination of the nervous system.

An example of this age-dependent relationship is that between brain damage and speech. The left cerebral hemisphere is the leading hemisphere for speech in the great majority of right-handed patients. A permanent defect results if the regions concerned with speech are irreversibly damaged in an adult. In young children, irreversible damage to either hemisphere may produce some speech loss which is usually neither complete nor permanent. After a period of time it may be impossible to detect any disturbance in language. This suggests that, in early childhood, the function of speech is represented bilaterally, with recovery of speech reflecting the ability of other areas of the cerebral hemispheres to assume that function. After the age of 5 years, speech begins to develop rigid lateralization so that permanent damage leaves some degree of permanent defect. Children show a similar ability to recover with greater ease than adults from the general effects of other forms of central nervous system damage, such as severe head injury or ischemic vascular lesions.

Evidence of neurologic dysfunction also depends upon the length of the interval which elapses following the insult to the nervous system. Immediately following spinal cord trauma, there may be a period in which spinal cord reflexes cannot be obtained. This is known as spinal shock, and lasts for variable periods in man to be followed by the appearance of autogenous spinal reflexes; it may be analogous to concussion injury to the brain.

The effect of disease on nervous function also varies according to the anatomic level of the nervous system which is involved. Organization of the nervous system becomes increasingly complex as one moves from peripheral nerve to spinal cord up through brainstem, diencephalon, and finally the cerebral hemispheres. The basic anatomic unit of the nervous system is the neuron, but the basic functional unit is the reflex and as one moves to higher functional levels in the nervous system, increasing numbers of anatomic systems and reflexes become involved. At low anatomic levels, the effect of structural damage can be predicted with some accuracy. For instance, if the ulnar nerve is cut at the elbow, the area of resulting motor and sensory loss varies little from one individual to the next. Lesions at specific locations in the spinal cord and brainstem also produce generally uniform although slightly less predictable and more modifiable results. The results of damage to the cerebral hemispheres show the greatest degree of variation among patients. However, even at this highest level, fairly accurate localization may be achieved, especially when sensory functions, such as vision, are involved.

It must not be forgotten that symptoms due to underlying structural changes may become manifest clinically by events in the patient's environment which in themselves do not produce any structural change. An example of this is seen following an abrupt change in the previously stable environment of a patient suffering from a dementing illness. If the patient's spouse suddenly dies he may find himself unable to cope with problems which previously had been quietly assumed by his wife. When this added responsibility is placed abruptly before a patient with diminishing powers of adaptation, his overall mental performance may suddenly deteriorate ("catastrophic reaction"), and he becomes unable to fend for himself, is brought to medical attention, and may thereafter require chronic care. Another example is the accentuation of physical signs which may be seen in a patient with Parkinsonism if he experiences a superadded depressive illness. It is thus readily apparent that although a recognizable structural disease process is present, environmental and psychologic factors may be crucial in determining the way in which the disease is manifest and the way in which the patient is able to adapt to it. With every patient, it is necessary to inquire carefully into relevant personal, family, vocational, and other factors, taking them all into account when drawing up a final formulation of the relative extent of underlying pathology.

LOCALIZATION OF NEUROLOGIC LESIONS

No single organ system can be considered in isolation when evaluating a disease process. Significant neurologic complications occur in 20 percent of all patients in a general hospital, an incidence which demands of all those dealing with such patients a working approach to the evaluation of neurologic symptoms. Although it is possible to go into considerable depth with many such patients, a highly sophisticated approach is generally unnecessary in reaching a conclusion about preliminary management. One of the first steps involved is that of determining the one or more locations in the central or peripheral nervous system where dysfunction is occurring. The following are some of the more common symptoms of cerebral, motor, or sensory dysfunction.

Cerebral Function

Cerebral lesions have a general deleterious effect on mental function irrespective of their location and depending in part upon their size, but, in addition, specific symptoms may be recognized pointing to involvement of focal regions of the cerebral hemispheres (Fig. 1.1). Frontal lobe damage produces changes in mood, such as euphoria, often accompanied by carelessness in behavior and dress. A grasp reflex may be elicited by stroking the palm of the contralateral hand, and, when undisturbed, the patient may lie clutching the bedclothes. Apraxia of gait and lack of control of urination are sometimes present. If the inferior frontal convolution of the left hemisphere (Broca's area) is involved, the patient may experience aphasia. Diffuse degenerative conditions involving the pre-central region will damage corticospinal fibers bilaterally, causing generalized hyperreflexia, dysarthria, and difficulty in swallowing (pseudobulbar palsy).

To perform a complex motor act, it is necessary first to formulate the idea of the act in one's mind, and then to carry it out. With damage to the parietal lobe, there may be an inability to formulate the idea (ideational apraxia) or the patient may be able to formulate a pattern of action which fails to be transmitted to the motor pathways (ideomotor apraxia). Apraxia is tested by having the patient demonstrate the use of objects such as a toothbrush or key or be asked to light a cigarette. The patient may be unable to dress himself, becoming muddled in attempts to put his arm through a sleeve ("Dressing apraxia"), indicating a lesion of the right parietal lobe. Another defect, common in lesions of the minor hemisphere, is an inability to copy simple arrangements of matches (constructional apraxia). If the angular gyrus of the dominant

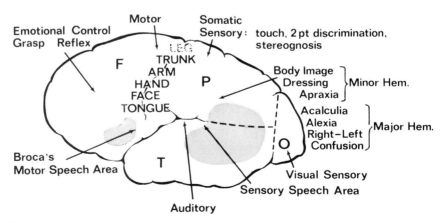

Figure 1.1. Schematic diagram of cerebral hemisphere showing major lobes and localization of certain functions. Although damage to certain areas may lead to specific symptoms, there are important relationships within and between the hemispheres so that the brain should be considered to function as a whole.

parietal lobe is involved, the patient experiences an inability to judge between right and left or to perform mathematical calculations and demonstrates an inability to identify individual fingers (finger agnosia). Damage to the parietal lobe or its connections may produce sensory inattention, so that when a patient is presented with equal stimuli given simultaneously to both sides of his body, he will ignore the one on the side of the body contralateral to the hemisphere lesion. Such a defect may be an important early sign of hemisphere damage.

Temporal lobe involvement is often associated with seizures, and these may begin with feelings of derealization or auditory, visual, or uncinate aurae. Visual field defects result from damage to the visual radiations. There may be an aphasic disturbance in the form of a naming disorder. Extensive bilateral temporal lobe involvement, particularly if the hippocampal gyri are included, can lead to profound memory disturbances. Amnestic syndromes also occur with lesions involving the mamillary bodies, fornix, and parts of the thalamus.

Lesions of the occipital lobes produce hemianopic field defects which may be incomplete, taking the form of visual inattention. Occipital seizures can produce sterotyped recurrent visual hallucinations, whereas changing, animated and more prolonged visual hallucinations suggest a toxic etiology.

Motor Function

For purposes of localization, motor function can be divided into two major divisions, the upper and the lower motor neuron. The term upper motor neuron is used to refer to the corticospinal (pyramidal) tract, which consists of axons arising primarily from the cells of the pre-central gyrus which then course downward through the internal capsule and brainstem. Most of these axons (about 80 percent) cross the midline at the lower aspect of the medulla. At the level of each motor cranial nerve, and each spinal segment, fibers leave the tract and synapse with motor neurons of the anterior horn as well as with interneurons at the base of the posterior horn. Damage to this suprasegmental system produces impairment or loss of movement, increased resistance of a limb to passive movement of a "clasp-knife" type, exaggerated deep tendon reflexes, and an extensor plantar response. The presence of these signs therefore alerts one to damage of the corticospinal system. Other signs may help localize the exact site of the lesion. For instance, a left hemiplegia and a right third nerve palsy would indicate a lesion in the right side of the midbrain. Signs of pyramidal damage may be modified by dysfunction of the extrapyramidal and vestibular systems which exert important influences on normal posture and movement (See Chapter 8).

The term lower motor neuron refers to the cell body in the motor nuclei of the brainstem or anterior horn of the spinal cord and its axon which terminates in relation to a number of muscle fibers. Damage at any point along the lower motor neruon can produce weakness, wasting, decreased resistance to passive movement (hypotonia), diminished reflexes, and spontaneous twitches of groups of muscle fibers (fasciculations) in the region supplied. Therefore, the presence of weakness in a hand and forearm with wasted muscles and reflex loss would direct attention to disease either of the anterior horn cells in the cervical portion of the spinal cord or along the course of the nerves issuing therefrom.

Sensory Function

The nature of disturbances of sensation also depends upon the anatomic level of the structural lesion. The types of sensation which may be altered with peripheral nerve damage include pain, heat and cold, light touch, position sense, and sense of vibration. Complete interruption of a major peripheral sensory nerve produces a relatively sharply demarcated area of loss of these sensations. With damage to the spinal cord the level of the lesion may be localized by careful sensory testing evaluating the same modalities. However, damage at higher levels in the nervous system interferes not only with the primary modes of sensation listed above, but may also cause a disturbance in more complicated sensory appreciation, such as discriminating two points from one point, localizing points touched, appreciating shape, form, texture, and weight, and recognizing by touch the nature of an object. Mild impairment of the primary forms of sensation with greater loss of more complicated types suggests damage at the level of the cerebral hemispheres.

FUNCTIONAL DISTURBANCE WITHOUT DEMONSTRABLE STRUCTURAL DISEASE

In the presence of damage to the nervous system, physical examination will reveal the extent of the disability and can provide important clues to localization. If damage is extensive, abnormal signs will be apparent to even the most inexperienced examiner, whereas considerable experience will be necessary to interpret correctly the significance of minor abnormalities. Frequently, however, patients will experience important symptoms of disordered function of the nervous system which are completely reversible, so that by the time such a patient is examined, no abnormality can be demonstrated. Common examples are a transient loss of consciousness or monocular blindness (amaurosis fugax). In such a situation, the examiner must rely entirely upon his interpretation of a carefully obtained history to make an accurate diagnosis and to reach a logical decision about additional investigation or treatment.

Seizures

Seizures provide a common example of a situation in which the patient experiences an alarming episode of disturbed central nervous system function, followed usually by a fairly rapid return to normal. Seizures may appear primarily as a manifestation of constitutional factors with no detectable underlying structural defect (idiopathic), or they may be a symptom of an associated static or progressive lesion (symptomatic). Seventy-five percent of patients with seizures are in the first category, and a decision to place the patient into one or the other group will influence the extent of investigation to be carried out in search of a demonstrable cause. The patient is occasionally unaware of the manifestations, and an eye-witness account by another observer may be essential.

Factors both general and specific operate in the production of seizures. The importance of age is demonstrated by the greatly lowered threshold to seizures of infants and children. Seizures frequently appear as a non-specific symptom in association with childhood systemic febrile illnesses, with as many as 5 to 7 percent of all children experiencing seizures prior to the age of 7 years. Seizures are secondary to significant underlying organic brain disease in only a very small minority of children.

Genetic factors result in an increased liability to seizures of patients who have one or more relatives with a seizure disorder. In some patients, such factors as hyperventilation, hypoglycemia, or specific afferent stimuli such as flickering lights may be required to precipitate a seizure, but the majority occur in the absence of detectable immediate cause. Some patients experience seizures only during sleep, a time when there is a tendency toward more synchronous neuronal activity.

Seizure discharges presumably result from periodic membrane instability in a group of neurons, leading to hyperactive and hypersynchronous neuronal firing. Membrane polarization is modified by various excitatory and inhibitory chemical agents and by the ionic balance across the cell membrane. In the presence of the appropriate biochemical milieu, hyperdepolarization occurs, leading to excessive neuronal firing. If this excessive discharge succeeds in obtaining adequate cellular recruitment, the discharge can spread along pre-existing neural pathways, interrupt normal central nervous system function, and lead to clinical sezures. Enhancement of synaptic transmission during repetitive stimulation (post-tetanic potentiation), contributes to the continuation of a seizure and is a feature diminished by anti-convulsant drugs. Diphenylhydantoin, a commonly used anti-convulsant drug, promotes an efflux of sodium from neurons. This tends to stabilize the hyperexcitability which may result from excessive stimulation or changes in the milieu which reduce the membrane sodium gradient. Synaptic post-tetanic potentiation is thereby reduced, limiting the spread of seizure discharge from a cortical focus. If seizure spread is extensive, there will be loss of consciousness, but if it remains localized, it may be manifest as a focal motor, sensory, or other type of limited seizure.

The anatomic basis of generalized seizure discharges remains largely unknown, but attention has been directed to the thalamus and reticular activating system as possible sites of seizure origin with spread occurring through thalamocortical pathways. Oscillation and feedback within such an anatomic system might explain the tonic and clonic features of a generalized seizure. Characteristic electrical patterns may be seen in the electroencephalogram in the interseizure period. Some recordings are characterized by generalized symmetrical discharges which project diffusely throughout the cerebral hemispheres (Fig. 1.2).

Although, by definition, structural change cannot be demonstrated in patients with idiopathic seizures, numerous neurologic diseases may have seizures as a symptom of organic central nervous system damage. Alterations in structure of neuronal dendrites have been reported in experimental models of epilepsy. Acquired cortical damage, for example trauma, may lead to the creation of standing negative potentials due to dendritic depolarization with the creation of an epileptogenic spike focus (Fig. 1.3). Such spike foci may lead to secondary activation of subcortical structures, so that the patient experiences a focal aura followed by a generalized seizure.

Vertigo

The complaint of dizziness or unsteadiness is another common neurologic symptom where, again, there may be marked episodic subjective disturbance without abnormalities at the time of physical examination. Symptoms of disease are often outside common experience and the patient may experience difficulty in describing his complaints. It is necessary to define as accurately as possible what the patient means by dizziness. In one patient it may represent intense repetitive attacks of vertigo (disordered orientation of the body in space), during which time the room suddenly appears to spin for a clearly defined period, accom-

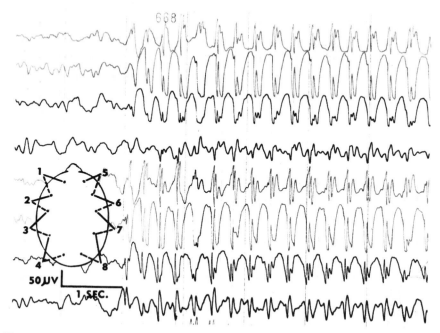

Figure 1.2. Electroencephalogram of 10 year old boy subject to absence attacks. Recording from left hemisphere. Note spontaneous abrupt and generalized onset of spike and wave discharge.

panied by tinnitus, nausea, and vomiting. The implication of such symptoms is quite different from those described by an anxious and depressed patient also complaining of dizziness, but who in fact experiences only a continuous sense of apprehension and fear that he may fall while walking. Although there may be little to find on examination, the presence or absence of other symptoms may enable one to decide about the mechansim of the symptoms. Anxious or depressed patients frequently complain of dizziness, but a sense of rotation is usually lacking and other characteristic psychogenic complaints are often present.

A vague sense of unsteadiness and, less frequently, a sense of true rotation may form part of the aura of cortical seizures or be part of an episode of transient cerebral ischemia. Ischemia of the brainstem is a more common cause of transient vertigo and may accompany neck movements which compromise flow through the vertebrobasilar or carotid systems (See Chapter 5).

Brainstem involvement with multiple sclerosis or neoplasms may produce episodic vertigo. Similar lesions involving the cerebellum, par-

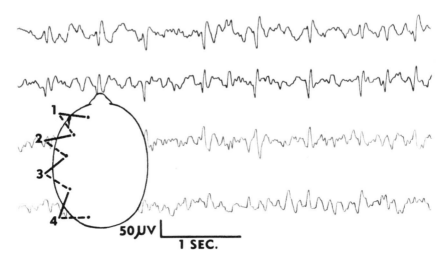

Figure 1.3. Interseizure record from a patient with spike focus in left frontal region. Patient experienced seizures characterized by turning of head and eyes to the right followed by loss of consciousness and generalized convulsion.

ticularly the flocculonodular lobe which has extensive vestibular connections, also cause vertigo.

Neoplastic, infective, or vascular lesions of the eighth nerve must be considered in a patient complaining of dizziness. Accompanying deafness and tinnitus are then often present. An acoustic neuroma is a common example (Fig. 10.7).

Labyrinthine disease is a common cause of vertigo and examples include otitis media, toxic drug effects, Ménière's syndrome, and vestibular neuronitis. The latter usually presents as a self-limited episode of vertigo which begins during or shortly after a respiratory or gastrointestinal infection, and may be an example of a parainfectious demyelinating disorder (See Chapter 6). Head injury may result in labyrinthine damage and resultant intense vertigo when the patient changes the position of his head. Nystagmus can often be observed when symptoms are present, and if this condition is not recognized, the patient may be dismissed as having neurotic complaints.

Vertigo, like seizures, is therefore a common complaint and one which may not be associated with physical signs. In evaluating this symptom, it is necessary to inquire into the function of all body systems, but with attention obviously focused toward the complaint. The presence or absence of associated symptoms will aid in localizing the complaint, and, in many patients, the diagnosis can be arrived at with the information obtained by careful history taking alone. In such situations, the physical examination serves only to confirm the diagnosis. It must not be forgotten that a combination of neurologic signs may be common to a number of different diseases and differentiation may be possible only by recording their mode of development. If there is doubt as to whether or not symptoms are due to physical or psychologic disease, signs obtained on examination may be essential in reaching a diagnosis.

Recent advances in radiologic, histologic, and biochemical techniques have been of great diagnostic value in selected patients. In the case of vertigo, new methods of auditory and labyrinthine testing assist in patient evaluation. However, such tests are required for only a minority of patients referred for neurologic evaluation. Patients in hospital with brain tumors and ruptured aneurysms are but a fraction of all those sent for an opinion concerning headache, dizziness, blackouts, or pain. For the majority, diagnosis will be carried out, and management decided upon, based primarily on a careful history and physical examination with only occasional need for extensive laboratory investigation.

REFERENCES

AJMONE MARSAN, C. A newly proposed classification of epileptic seizures: neurophysiological basis. Epilepsia 6:275, 1965.

COATS, A. C. Vestibular neuronitis. Acta Otolaryng. (Stockholm) Suppl. 251, 1969.

FRANTZEN, E., LENNOX-BUCHTHAL, M., NYGAARD, A., AND STENE, J. Genetic study of febrile convulsions. Neurology (Minneap.) 20:909, 1970.

HOLMES, SIR GORDON. Introduction to Clinical Neurology. 3rd edition. E. & S. Livingstone, Ltd., Edinburgh, 1968.

JASPER, H. H., WARD, A. A., JR., AND POPE, A. Basic Mechanisms of the Epilepsies. Little, Brown & Co., Boston, 1969.

KILOH, L. G., AND OSSELTON, J. W. Clinical Electroencephalography. 2nd edition. Butterworth & Co., Ltd., London, 1966.

MATHEWS, W. B. Practical Neurology. Blackwell Scientific Publications, Ltd., Oxford, 1963.

MAYER-GROSS, W., SLATER, E., AND ROTH, M. Clinical Psychiatry. 3rd edition. Cassell & Co., Ltd., London, 1969.

SCHMIDT, R. P., AND WILDER, B. J. Epilepsy. Contemporary Neurology Series Monograph No. 2. F. A. Davis Co., Philadelphia, 1968.

WEISS, P. One plus one does not equal two. In The Neurosciences. A Study Program. Ed. by G. C. Quarton, T. Melnechuk, and F. O. Schmitt. The Rockefeller University Press, New York, 1967.

WOLFSON, R. J. (Ed). The Vestibular System and Its Diseases. University of Pennsylvania Press, Philadelphia, 1966.

2

CELLULAR REACTIONS TO INJURY

INTRODUCTION

The reactions of the nervous system to injury are not different in principle from those of the rest of the body. Basic processes such as inflammation and repair, degeneration, and neoplasia occur in the brain in much the same fashion as in other organs and tissues, although occasionally the resemblance is obscured by differences in terminology and by the brain's architectural complexity.

For the purpose of understanding its reaction to disease, the nervous system may conveniently be thought of as composed of two tissue populations. The connective tissues, blood vessels, and phagocytic cells constitute a population shared with the remainder of the body. The neurons and macroglia are unique to the nervous system. They have distinctive morphologic and functional characteristics, as well as a specific and limited range of pathologic reactions, a knowledge of which is the basis of an understanding of neuropathology.

A major limiting factor in the study of neuropathology is the inherent complexity of the nervous system (Figs. 2.1, 2.2, 2.3). It is impossible to analyze in detail either the structure of the normal brain or the distribution of pathologic changes in more than a very superficial fashion with presently available techniques. The human brain contains about 20 billion neurons, each of which makes or receives as many as several hundred or occasionally several thousand synapses, some a meter or more from the cell of origin. Neurons are themselves far from being a homogeneous population. Specific nuclei and specific cortical and brainstem areas not only have distinctive morphologic and biochemical characteristics, but also demonstrate very different susceptibilities to injurious agents. In a few areas of the brain, for example the cerebellar cortex, there is a good deal known about the details of synaptic organization and biochemical characteristics of the neurons, but in most regions only an intriguing glimpse of the general anatomic pattern and of neuronal interactions has thus far emerged. It is not surprising, then,

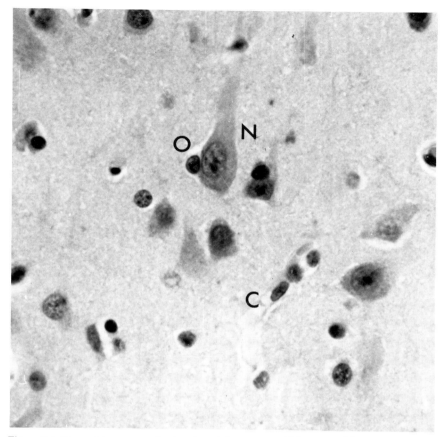

Figure 2.1. Normal human cerebral cortex. A large pyramidal neuron (*N*) is readily identified by virtue of its shape, abundant cytoplasm, large vesicular nucleus, and prominent nucleolus. There are several spherical dense nuclei of glial cells in the photograph; their cell bodies are inconspicuous. The processes of one satellite oligodendroglial cell (*O*) are apparent because of artifactual swelling. A small capillary (*C*) is present. The finely granular background (the neuropil) is composed of the closely packed processes of the various cell types. (Hematoxylin-phloxine-saffron, × 275)

to find that pathologic study of the brain often fails to provide adequate answers to questions posed by the clinical picture. On the other hand, the comparatively crude techniques available for clinical assessment of cerebral function in humans may often fail to provide the appropriate questions.

An additional feature affecting the analysis of neurologic disease is that of localization of function in specific nuclei and tracts. For example,

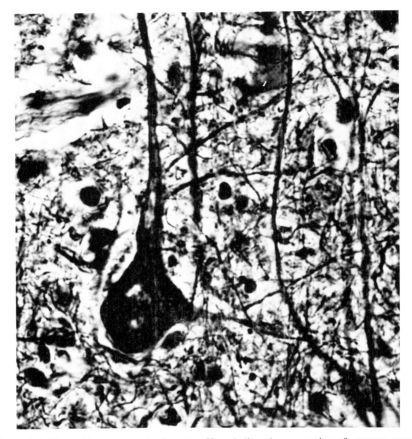

Figure 2.2. Normal human cerebral cortex. Use of silver impregnation of neurons, axons, and dendrites renders visible some of the complexity of the neural network. Although glial nuclei are stained their processes are not. A few intracellular neurofibrils (not well-preserved) are seen in the apical dendrite close to the neuronal cell body. (Bielschowsky, × 500)

a small infarct in the frontal region of a hemisphere will have radically different consequences for the patient than will a similar lesion in the lateral medulla, although the etiologic factors and progression of tissue changes are essentially the same in the two locations.

In general, analysis of a neurologic case involves two distinct steps—first, to determine *where* the lesion is, based on knowledge of neuro-anatomy and neurophysiology, and secondly, on the basis of all the available information, to deduce *what* the lesion is. Some disease processes, for example infarcts or infections, may occur essentially anywhere, whereas other entities have a highly selective anatomic pattern

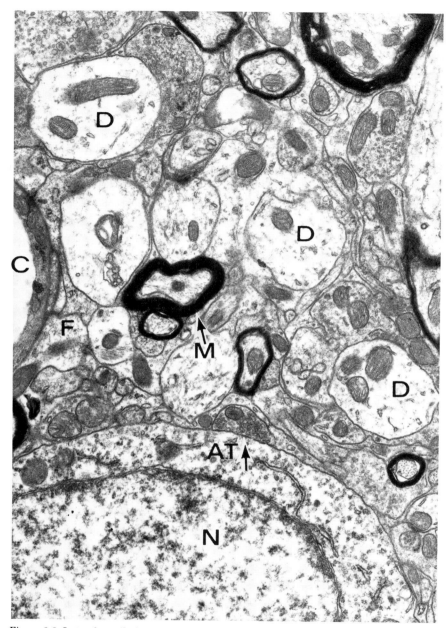

Figure 2.3. Lateral vestibular nucleus, rat. A small neuron (*N*) has rather scant cytoplasm containing numerous free ribosomes, endoplasmic reticulum, and a mitochondrion. An axon terminal (*AT*) containing synaptic vesicles lies against the neuronal membrane. A few of the processes are readily identified as axons by virtue of their myelin sheaths (*M*). Around a capillary (*C*) are several astrocytic foot processes (*F*). Several of the large relatively clear processes (*D*) are dendrites, many of which are in contact with axonal terminals. The neuropil is almost totally occupied by the tightly packed cell processes; there is very little extracellular space. (Electron micrograph, × 14,500)

of involvement, a knowledge of which is of fundamental importance in reaching a correct diagnosis.

NEURONAL REACTIONS IN DISEASE

Neuronal abnormalities are the cornerstone of neuropathology in that most (but by no means all) injurious agents act primarily on nerve cells.

There are two fundamental principles involved in neuronal reactions:

1. Lost neurons are not replaced. Humans at birth have essentially a full complement of nerve cells which behave as a fixed post-mitotic population.

2. Neurons are metabolically very active; they require a continuous supply of oxygen, glucose, and other metabolites, and are in general very sensitive to alterations in electrolyte levels, pH, etc., in their environment.

As with other cell populations, both lethal and non-lethal neuronal changes occur, and some are more easily identified than others by the pathologist. For example, mild changes such as neuronal swelling and dispersal of endoplasmic reticulum (Nissl substance), probably equivalent to cloudy swelling and loss of basophilia in damaged hepatic and other cells, are often difficult to interpret in autopsy material since they may occur as agonal phenomena or as post-mortem artifacts as well as in a number of pathologic circumstances. In experimental material where adequate controls are possible and good fixation is obtained, these changes can be highly significant, particularly when correlated with electron microscopic evidence of abnormalities in the various cytoplasmic organelles.

On the other hand, *loss* of neurons is highly convincing evidence of disease. Unfortunately, quantitative assessment of neuronal or axonal populations is a difficult and time-consuming task and is not yet routinely practical; a diffuse loss of up to 30 percent or more of cortical neurons may easily go undetected. Presumably, automated cell-counting methods will eventually be developed to make this sort of assessment feasible. Total or patchy depletion is more easily recognized. In addition, neuronal loss is almost invariably accompanied by astrocytic proliferation which serves as a very useful marker of previous damage.

Recent neuronal *necrosis* is readily recognized (Fig. 2.4). As in other cells, nuclei become pyknotic and fragmented, the cell bodies become shrunken, angular, and more eosinophilic, and, in addition, neurofibrils and Nissl substance are lost. These changes are best seen in large neurons in areas of recent infarction, but anoxia, hypoglycemia, viral infections, trauma, etc., produce a similar appearance. The necrotic cells commonly incite a phagocytic response.

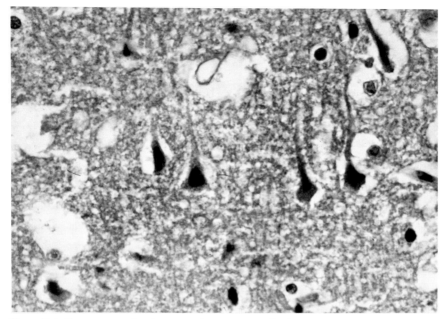

Figure 2.4. Recent necrosis of neurons. Infarct of cerebral cortex, 24 hours old. Neurons are shrunken, irregular, and angular in outline, with nuclear pyknosis. There is also marked edema; processes in the neuropil are swollen and more easily seen than in the normal. (Hematoxylin-eosin (HE), × 350)

Atrophy of neurons occurs in a number of "degenerative" slowly progressive disease states, and may also occur as an age-related phenomenon. Atrophic neurons appear smaller than normal; nuclei appear abnormally dense, and lipofuscin pigment accumulates in abnormal amounts. The axons and dendrites, normally difficult to distinguish in routine stains, become eosinophilic and irregular in shape and stand out against the paler neuropil. Presumably, these cells will eventually die, leaving behind a marker in the form of some degree of glial proliferation.

Neuronal *inclusions* are found in a number of cirumstances, and are often of major diagnostic importance to the pathologist. For example, in a number of inborn errors of sphingolipid metabolism, the cytoplasm becomes greatly distended with distinctive lipid-laden lysosomal derivatives. In several viral infections including Herpes simplex encephalitis and rabies (Fig. 2.5), characteristic inclusion bodies occur in infected cells. Parkinson's disease and idiopathic familial myoclonus epilepsy are both associated with large spherical intracytoplasmic accumulations containing fibrillar material of uncertain nature, referred to as Lewy

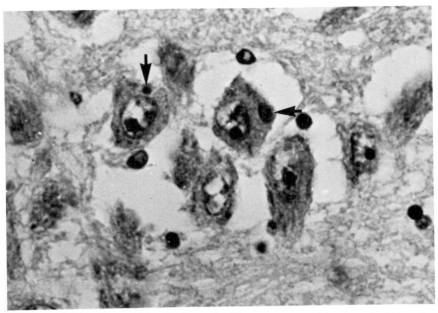

Figure 2.5. Rabies. Pyramidal cells from the hippocampus contain characteristic cyto-plasmic inclusions (*arrows*), known as Negri bodies. (HE, × 575)

bodies (Fig. 9.11) and Lafora bodies, respectively. These and other neuronal inclusions are discussed under the appropriate headings. In addition, several types of nuclear and cytoplasmic inclusions of unknown significance or nature are often found in certain cell groups in routine autopsies and are occasionally misconstrued as evidence of disease by the unwary examiner.

Neurofibrillary degeneration is the accumulation of coarse whorls or skeins of filamentous material in the cytoplasm of the cell body (Fig. 9.5) and dendrites, best seen with silver impregnation or by electron microscopy. The coarse fibrils seen by light microscopy are composed of bundles of fine (100 Å) twisted filaments arranged in parallel arrays. This change is conspicuous in Alzheimer's disease but also occurs in other degenerative diseases and some virus infections. The source of the filaments is uncertain; they may be derived from neurofilaments, but they have a somewhat different structure. This change is discussed further in Chapter 9.

AXONAL REACTIONS

Much of the mass of the nervous system is composed of axons, either densely intertwined with dendrites and cell bodies or running in parallel as the great fiber tracts of the brain and spinal cord and in the peripheral nerves. While many axons are very short, others are a meter or more in length. The maintenance of a cylinder of cytoplasm 3 or 4 feet in length and only a few microns in diameter presents some very special problems which are not yet completely solved. Presumably, their shape is determined by their content of microtubules (usually called neurotubules in neurons) and neurofilaments. They depend on their cell of origin for most or all of their enzymes and other proteins and for other metabolites as well, and a continuous centripetal flow can be demonstrated. Glucose, oxygen, and electrolytes are extracted from the local environment throughout their length, and other metabolites including those involved in chemical transmission of impulses are in part transported directly across the axonal membrane.

In 1850, A. V. Waller found that when the hypoglossal nerve was cut, the portions of axons distal to the section became fragmented and disappeared in a few days (Figs 2.6, 2.7). This phenomenon, now referred

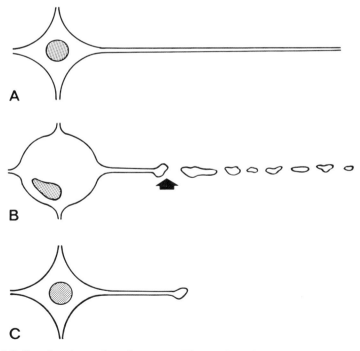

Figure 2.6. Reaction to section of an axon. The portion of the axon beyond the section (*arrow*) undergoes fragmentation (*B*) and eventual lysis (*C*). A retraction ball forms at the end of the proximal portion, and persists for some time. The cell body swells, with peripheral migration of its nucleus during the acute phase (*B*).

to as *Wallerian degeneration*, is an invariable occurrence in that portion of an axon separated from its cell body in both the central and peripheral nervous systems. It is used extensively by neuroanatomists in tracing fiber tracts, and is also a conspicuous feature of naturally occurring lesions in which axons are interrupted at some point in their course. If the axon is myelinated, the sheath also undergoes fragmentation and is subsequently digested by macrophages (Figs. 2.8, 2.9) and, in peripheral nerves, by the Schwann cells themselves.

The fate of the proximal axonal segment and of the cell body is variable and depends on the specific population of cells involved. In lesions of many central tracts, the cells of origin undergo slowly progressive atrophy and finally disappear after months or years. In other tracts there may be attempted regrowth of the severed axons, but this invariably fails after a few days. Successful functional regeneration of severed axons in the central nervous system of mammals has not been accomplished despite much experimental effort, and does not occur in humans.

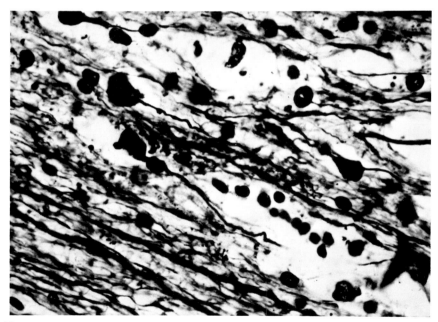

Figure 2.7. Axonal fragmentation in cerebral white matter following mechanical disruption as the result of shearing forces generated in an automobile accident. Several axons exhibit marked beading and irregularity; in some instances the continuity of the axonal "balls" with the normal portions of axons is evident. Compare with Figure 2.6. (Bodian, × 550)

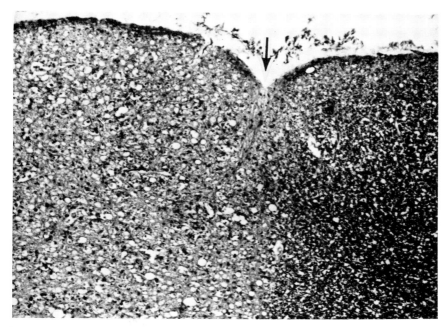

Figure 2.8. Wallerian degeneration, cervical spinal cord. The spinal cord had been severed at the 6th thoracic segment several weeks previously. An *arrow* marks the posteromedial fissure between the gracile and cuneate fasciculi. The cuneate fasciculus, on the *right*, is not involved since entry of its axons into the cord is above this level. The gracile fasciculus, on the *left*, the axons of which were interrupted by the lesion, has undergone marked loss of myelinated fibers, and thus appears pale and vacuolated. (Luxol fast blue-hematoxylin-eosin (LFB-HE), × 50)

In peripheral nerves, however, the situation is entirely different. Vigorous sprouting occurs at the proximal stump, and if the cut ends of the nerve are in good apposition, the sprouts quickly make contact with the distal segment. Schwann cells in the distal segment proliferate to form long cylindrical aggregates along which the newly formed axons grow at the rate of about 1 mm per day until they reach muscle or a sensory location; myelination subsequently occurs. If the cut ends are separated or scar tissue is interposed, the proliferating axons and fibrous tissue form a tangled lump referred to as a traumatic neuroma.

The functional success of peripheral nerve regeneration is highly variable. If there is a significant gap, many axons will be lost in the neuroma. Motor axons may end up in the skin or in the wrong muscle groups or sensory axons in muscle where they serve no useful function. A rather spectacular example of aberrant regeneration is occasionally seen following facial nerve injuries when parasympathetic salivatory fibers re-

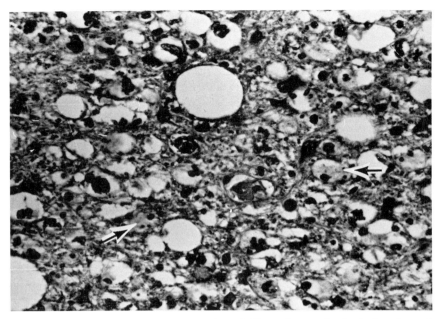

Figure 2.9. Wallerian degeneration, spinal cord. From the gracile fasciculus shown in Figure 2.8. Myelin sheaths have broken down, leaving irregular clumps of lipid; numerous macrophages (*arrows*) are present. (LFB-HE, × 350)

innervate the lacrimal gland, resulting in profuse lacrimation at meal-time—so-called "crocodile tears." However, careful surgical reconstruction of severed peripheral nerves may be followed by satisfactory return of function.

Three additional features of axonal interruption merit mention. "Axonal reaction" or "central chromatolysis" is seen in some cell bodies, notably the motor cranial nuclei and anterior horn cells, in the weeks following axonal section (Fig. 2.10). The cell swells, the nucleus migrates to the periphery, the nucleoli enlarge, Nissl bodies become dispersed, and lysosomal enzyme activity is increased. This reaction is associated with greatly increased nucleic acid and protein synthesis, undoubtedly related to concomitant axonal regeneration. The changes are easily seen histologically and thus form a useful neuroanatomic tool in those systems in which it occurs.

If the optic nerve is interrupted, the axonal endings in the lateral geniculate body undergo Wallerian degeneration. During the next several months, the cells of the geniculate body undergo atrophy and finally are lost—*trans-synaptic degeneration.* This occurs as well in other circumstances where neurons are deprived of all or most of their afferent connections. *Retrograde trans-synaptic degeneration* is the opposite phenomenon. After neurons are lost, cells whose axons had synapsed with them may gradually be lost. These "chain reactions" greatly complicate the analysis of long-standing pathologic processes where it becomes a difficult matter to know which of the involved interconnected nuclei and tracts were the site of the primary lesion.

REACTIONS OF GLIA

The glia ("glue") are a mixed population of cells of two basic types: the neuroectodermal derivatives—astrocytes, oligodendroglia, and ependyma, and the mesodermal microglia. The neuroectodermal cells are supportive and nutritive elements, while microglia are phagocytic cells of the histiocyte series.

Astrocytes

In the normal brain there are two populations of astrocytes. Fibrous astrocytes are those containing in their cytoplasmic processes arrays of long 100 Å filaments which probably provide some degree of mechanical strength. These are particularly numerous in the subpial (Fig.

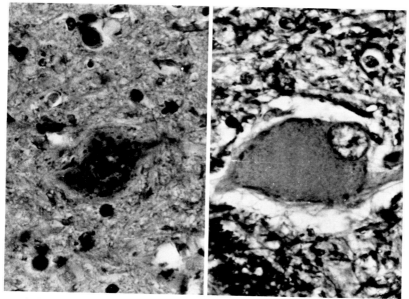

Figure 2.10. A (left): normal motor neuron of hypoglossal nucleus. *B (right):* central chromatolysis following destruction of the hypoglossal nerve at the base of the skull by extension of a nasopharyngeal carcinoma. (A and B: LFB-HE, × 500)

2.11) and subependymal tissues and are widely distributed through white matter and many of the nuclei. Protoplasmic astrocytes are morphologically similar cells which have few or no intracellular fibrils, and which predominate in layers two to five of the cerebral cortex and in the striatum. One or more of the numerous branching processes of both types end in relation to capillary basement membranes around which they form virtually continuous sheaths thought to play a role in metabolic transport across the blood-brain barrier (Fig. 2.3).

Astrocytes are considerably more resistant to anoxia and ischemia than neurons; if killed, they show the expected nuclear and cytoplasmic features of necrosis.

The principal reaction of astrocytes is that of gliosis or glial scar formation, a reaction seen in relation to most destructive neural lesions of more than a few days' duration. In contrast to neurons, astrocytes are capable of vigorous proliferation. Their cell bodies usually undergo considerable hypertrophy at the same time and become readily visible by light microscopy—the so-called gemistocytic ("fat") astrocytes, an im-

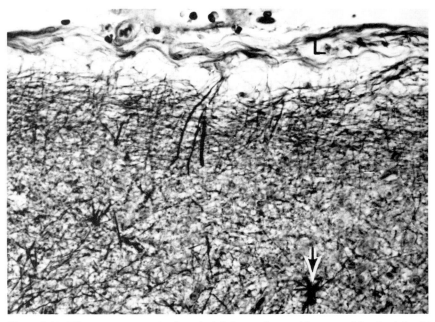

Figure 2.11. Fibrous astrocytes in the subpial tissue of normal human midbrain stained in a fashion to show their processes, which form a dense feltwork below the pial surface. Origin of the processes from a cell body is occasionally in the plane of section (*arrow*). Collagen fibers are present in the adjacent leptomeninges (*L*). (Phosphotungstic acid-hematoxylin (PTAH), × 300)

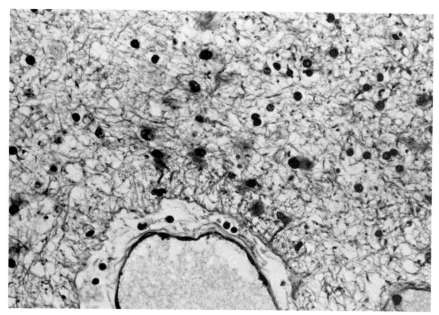

Figure 2.12. Astrocytic hypertrophy and hyperplasia near the edge of an old cerebral infarct. Several plump (gemistocytic) astrocytes are seen. Since other tissue elements were destroyed, the interwoven astrocytic processes making up the glial scar are easily seen in routine stains. A vein, the Virchow-Robin space, and its delimiting pial-glial interface are clearly seen, and some astrocytic processes are observed to end in relation to the pia. (HE, × 130)

portant marker of an astrocytic reaction (Fig. 2.12). Reactive protoplasmic astocytes develop abundant intracellular fibrils and are thus converted to the fibrous form. A glial scar is therefore formed of the densely interwoven cytoplasmic processes of fibrous astrocytes. It must be emphasized that the moderate firmness and mechanical strength of a glial scar are due to the intracellular fibrils; astroctyes do not form collagen. Occasionally, as around a hemorrhage or abscess, fibroblasts from adjacent vessels or meninges also participate in the repair response, in which case a mixed fibroglial scar is formed.

Astroglial proliferation is almost always secondary to destructive lesions of either neurons or myelin (Fig. 2.13). However, a few exceptions to this general principle exist; in chronic hepatic failure, and occasionally in other metabolic derangements, there may be considerable proliferation of protoplasmic astrocytes of the putamen, caudate nucleus, and cerebral cortex without morphologic evidence of neuronal damage. The astrocytic nuclei are usually markedly enlarged and irregu-

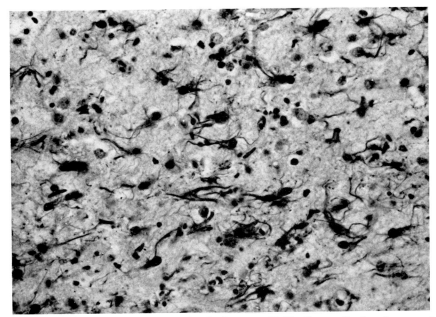

Figure 2.13. Astrocytic proliferation. Cerebral cortex, Pick's disease. Profound neuronal loss has been followed by marked gliosis, a common reaction in a number of such diseases. (PTAH, × 350)

lar in shape, and appear vacuolated as a result of intranuclear glycogen accumulation (Type II cells of Alzheimer) (Fig. 4.10). The cytoplasm remains inconspicuous, but may contain fine greenish-yellow granules of unknown nature. The mechanism of this remarkable, apparently primary astrocytosis is unknown.

Oligodendroglia

There are two distinct and probably unrelated populations of oligodendroglia—the neuronal satellite cells which partially ensheathe neurons and which are notable for their conspicuous ribosomal content, and the myelin-forming interfascicular oligodendroglia, by far the most numerous type of cell in the central nervous system. The function of the perineuronal oligodendroglia remains an enigma; they may have a nutritive function with respect to the neuron, and some have suggested that they play a role in long-term memory in relation to their synthesis of ribonucleic acid and protein.

Oligodendroglia of both types are quite sensitive to injury, but somewhat less so than neurons. They are prone to develop cytoplasmic swelling (hydropic change) so readily that it is present in almost all autopsy tissue and is not a useful indication of disease (Fig. 2.14).

In areas where myelin is destroyed (see below), oligodendroglia are reduced in number or disappear. In their place is an increase in astrocytes. It has been proposed that under certain circumstances oligodendroglia may in fact be converted to astrocytes and thus participate in glial scar formation.

In chronic disease with neuronal atrophy, there may be proliferation of perineuronal oligodendrocytes ("satellitosis"), the significance of which is unknown.

Ependyma

The ependymal lining of the ventricles may be destroyed by viral and bacterial infections, or may be stretched and broken by enlargement of the ventricles in hydrocephalus. Ependymal cells appear to have rather limited powers of regeneration and gaps are usually filled by astrocytic scar tissue which gives the surfaces a finely textured granular appearance, loosely referred to as "granular ependymitis" (Figs. 2.15,

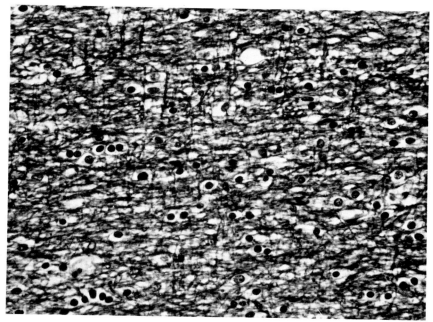

Figure 2.14. Normal white matter. Myelin sheaths appear as irregular dark lines or small cylinders; rows of interfascicular oligodendroglia shows "halos" around the nuclei, the result of cytoplasmic swelling, a common artifact in autopsy material. (LFB-HE, × 325)

2.16). Nests of ependymal cells buried beneath the surface by the astrocytic proliferation frequently form small rosettes resembling, in section, miniature spinal central canals.

Microglia

During intra-uterine life, a small number of cells of the reticuloendothelial system invade the developing nervous system and persist as

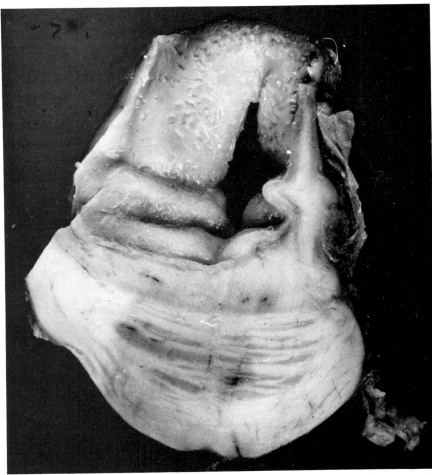

Figure 2.15. Granular "ependymitis." Male, 14 years, severely hydrocephalic as a result of meningeal fibrosis. The upper end of the 4th ventricle is markedly dilated and distorted, with extensive old ulceration of the ependyma. Section at the level of upper pons, looking rostrally. Note also the bilateral atrophy of corticospinal tracts secondary to cerebral atrophy.

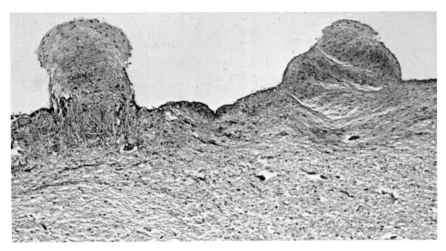

Figure 2.16. Granular "ependymitis." Previous ependymal ulceration with humps of astrocytic scar tissue protruding through the gaps above the level of the ependyma. (HE, × 50)

meningeal and perivascular phagocytes, and, in the parenchyma, as microglia. In disease processes, these cells respond by proliferation and hypertrophy as do histiocytes or macrophages elsewhere in the body, and are the principal phagocytic element in most disease states.

It is clear that in inflammatory lesions macrophages are derived from two sources, from the microglia already present in the area and, more importantly, from circulating monocytes which have migrated through the vessel walls under the influence of chemotactic stimuli.

Microglia are inconspicuous in the normal brain. Their cytoplasm is markedly attenuated and finely branched (Fig. 2.17), and, as with other glial cell processes cannot be distinguished easily from the background of the neuropil unless special stains are used. Under some circumstances, particularly in gray matter, hypertrophy leads to the formation of "rod cells"—large bipolar histiocytes (Fig. 2.18). More commonly, the cells become rounded to the more conventional configuration of macrophages, and as they accumulate phagocytosed and partly digested material, notably lipids, the cytoplasm becomes quite abundant and reticulated, an appearance referred to as "gitter cells" or "compound granular corpuscles" in the older literature (Fig. 2.19).

Recently dead neurons, particularly in viral infections, frequently attract a cluster of macrophages which surround and phagocytose the dead cell (Fig. 2.20). This phenomenon is referred to as neuronophagia.

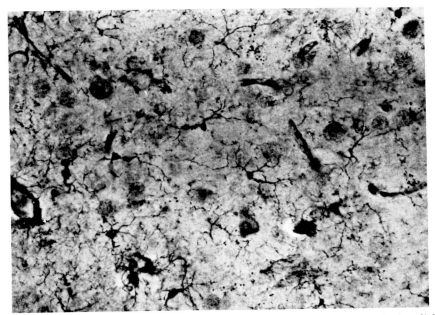

Figure 2.17. Normal microglia, rodent cortex. The fine branching processes of microglial cells are readily distinguished in this silver impregnation. (Hortega, × 500)

REACTIONS OF MYELIN SHEATHS

Although myelin sheaths are the highly specialized, attenuated cell membranes of oligodendroglia and Schwann cells, their reactions in disease are of sufficient importance to consider them separately.

Breakdown of myelin is a prominent and easily recognized pathologic change in a wide range of disease processes. There are at least five mechanisms whereby this may occur.

1. In destructive lesions, such as infarcts, in which both neural and glial elements have been killed, the myelin sheaths share in the process of dissolution of the destroyed tissue.

2. In any process which results in loss of axons, the corresponding myelin sheaths are also lost. This is best seen in Wallerian degeneration, in both the central and peripheral nervous systems, where the damaged fiber tracts or nerve fascicles can be traced using stains to demonstrate either loss of myelin or, in recent lesions, myelin breakdown products.

3. Myelin sheaths (presumably the oligodendroglia or Schwann cells) are primarily affected in several toxic and metabolic disturbances. In areas of chronic cerebral edema, widespread demyelination occurs.

Following carbon monoxide exposure, some patients develop widespread cerebral demyelination. Diabetes mellitus and chronic uremia are associated with primary demyelination of peripheral nerves. Diphtheria toxin also primarily damages Schwann cells and peripheral myelin.

4. In the primary demyelinating diseases of unknown etiology, including multiple sclerosis, there is considerable evidence that one or more components of the myelin sheaths are selectively and specifically destroyed. This is discussed in Chapter 6.

5. In the leukodystrophies, a group of inherited diseases known or thought to be inborn errors of metabolism, there is defective myelin formation in the developing brain, and in some, breakdown of previously formed myelin as well.

In the first two groups, it is apparent that the demyelination is merely secondary to other factors. In the last three, where there is little or no primary neuronal or axonal damage and no loss of tissue integrity, the term "primary demyelination" may be applied.

Regardless of the cause, myelin breakdown in both the central and peripheral nervous system follows a similar pattern. First, the sheaths

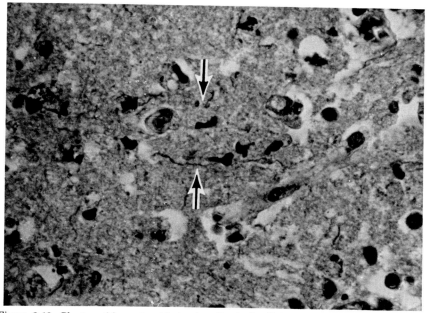

Figure 2.18. Cluster of hypertrophied microglia (rod cells) in an early lesion of Herpes simplex encephalitis (*arrows*). (HE, × 450)

become irregular in contour; the lamellae become separated, folded, and arranged in irregular and abnormal configurations. As structural integrity is lost, the lipoprotein material coalesces as numerous small or large globules which are taken up and digested by macrophages and in peripheral nerves, by Schwann cells. Some of the complex lipid is transformed to neutral fat, readily demonstrated by suitable stains in frozen sections (Figs. 2.21, 2.22). In the central nervous system, oligodendroglia disappear, and gliosis occurs. Schwann cell proliferation and endoneurial fibrosis are common findings in demyelinated peripheral nerves. Myelin in the central nervous system is not known to be

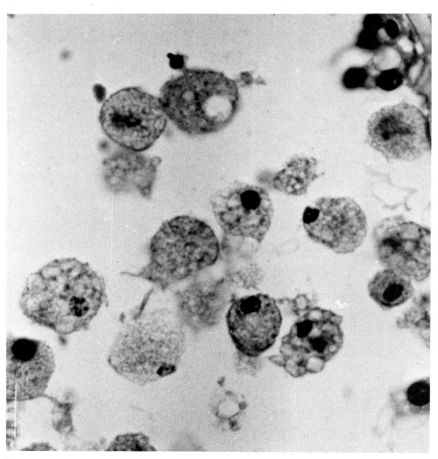

Figure 2.19. Macrophages loaded with lipid in the cavity of an old cerebral infarct. (HE, × 600)

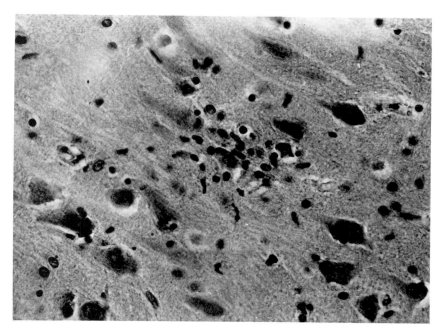

Figure 2.20. Neuronophagia of a recently dead neuron by a cluster of macrophages. Encephalitis, probably of viral origin. (HE, × 350)

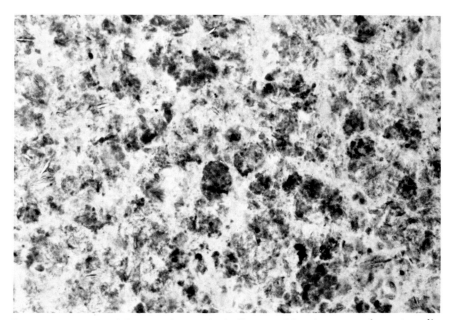

Figure 2.21. Lipid breakdown products, principally neutral fats, in an area of recent myelin damage in multiple sclerosis. Most of the lipid is in clusters, corresponding to hypertrophied macrophages such as seen in Figure 2.19. (Frozen section, oil red O (ORO), × 135)

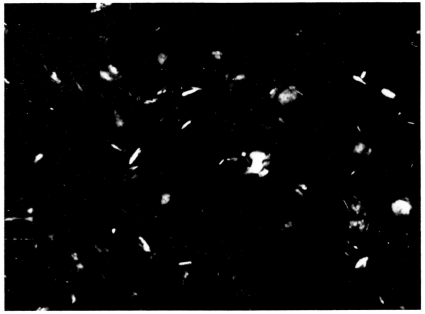

Figure 2.22. Same field as Figure 2.21, under polarized light. The needle-like crystals are cholesterol esters derived from the myelin sheaths. (Frozen section, ORO, × 135)

replaced except in certain experimental circumstances. Remyelination occurs much more readily in the peripheral nerves.

In several of the toxic and metabolic peripheral neuropathies, peripheral nerves show multiple foci of demyelination along the course of relatively intact axons interspersed among normally myelinated or remyelinated segments. In this reaction, referred to as segmental demyelination, each demyelinated region represents damage to one or several contiguous Schwann cells. Although the axon may continue to conduct impulses, the loss of saltatory conduction in the demyelinated segments produces marked slowing of conduction velocity as measured clinically.

REFERENCES

BLINKOV, S. M., AND GLEZER, I. I. The Human Brain in Figures and Tables. A Quantitative Handbook. Basic Books, Inc., New York, 1968.

FIELDS, W. S., AND WILLIS, W. D., JR. (Eds). The Cerebellum in Health and Disease. Warren H. Green, Inc., St. Louis, 1970.

GRAY, E. G., AND GUILLERY, R. W. Synaptic morphology in the normal and degenerating nervous system. Int. Rev. Cytol. 19:111, 1966.

LAMPERT, P. W. A comparative electron microscopic study of reactive, degenerating, regenerating, and dystrophic axons. J. Neuropath. Exp. Neurol. 26:345, 1967.

MENDELL, J. R., AND MARKESBERY, W. R. Neuronal intracytoplasmic hyaline inclusions. J. Neuropath. Exp. Neurol. 30:233, 1971.

NATHANIEL, E. J. H., AND PEASE, D. C. Degenerative changes in rat dorsal roots during Wallerian degeneration. J. Ultrastruct. Res. 9:511, 1963.

PETERS, A., PALAY, S. L., AND WEBSTER, H. De F. The Fine Structure of the Nervous System: the Cells and Their Processes. Hoeber Medical Division, Harper and Row, Publishers, New York, 1970.

POSER, C. M. Diseases of the myelin sheath. *In* Pathology of the Nervous System. Ed. by J. Minckler. McGraw-Hill Book Co., New York, 1968.

RAMÓN Y CAJAL, S. Degeneration and Regeneration of the Nervous System. Oxford University Press, London, 1928.

ROBERTS, E. D. P. DE, AND CARRERA, R. (Eds). Biology of neuroglia. *In* Progress in Brain Research, Vol. 15. Elsevier Press, Inc., New York, 1965.

ROSENBLUTH, J. Functions of glial cells. *In* The Central Nervous System: Some Experimental Models of Neurological Disease. Ed. by O. T. Bailey and D. E. Smith. The Williams & Wilkins Co., Baltimore, 1968.

TERRY, R. D. Neuronal fibrous protein in human pathology. J. Neuropath. Exp. Neurol. 30:8, 1971.

3

CEREBROSPINAL FLUID AND INTRA-CRANIAL FLUID DYNAMICS

The craniospinal cavity may be regarded as an almost rigid bony box completely filled by tissues, cerebrospinal fluid, and circulating blood. Although the rigidity of the coverings serves to protect the nervous system from mechanical injury, it may become a major liability; since the volume of the system is fixed, any additional intracranial mass such as blood or edema fluid is poorly tolerated. Under appropriate circumstances, as little as 80 ml of rapidly added volume will raise the intracranial pressure to a level incompatible with life. Increased intracranial pressure with the resulting circulatory disturbances and shifts of cerebral tissue within the cranium form the final common pathway to death in numerous diseases. Clinical recognition of elevated intracranial pressure is one of the most important steps in evaluation of a neurologic patient, and the associated symptoms and signs should be familiar to all medical practitioners.

INCREASED INTRACRANIAL PRESSURE

Intracranial pressure may be elevated by an increase in the volume of the brain or of cerebrospinal fluid as a result of disease, the accumulation of any extraneous material such as blood or pus, or vasodilatation. The clinical and pathologic effects are dependent upon the rate and height of the pressure elevation and, if focal, the location of the causative lesion.

Some compensation occurs as an intracranial lesion expands, but it is limited and may in itself be harmful. The ventricles contain about 40 ml of fluid and another few ml are in the subarachnoid space surrounding the brain. As cerebral mass increases, cerebrospinal fluid is displaced into the blood stream. The ventricles are compressed, sometimes to mere slits, and as the subarachnoid space is compressed, the brain flattens against the dura, and sulci are obliterated.

The elevated pressure also reduces the intracranial blood volume by compression of the venous and capillary beds. Protective reflexes usually attempt to maintain cerebral perfusion by producing elevation of the systemic blood pressure (the Cushing response), an important clinical sign of rising intracranial pressure. As cerebral perfusion is diminished, ischemia results and in turn leads to additional cerebral edema and further elevation of intracranial pressure. Finally the intracranial pressure approaches the arterial pressure and cerebral circulation stops.

In the case of slowly expanding lesions such as slow-growing tumors, pressure atrophy occurs in adjacent brain tissue. The white matter near a focal lesion is more susceptible to atrophy than is the cortex. The damaged tissue may give rise to focal signs and symptoms. In general, slowly expanding masses are better tolerated than rapid accumulations, and may reach much greater dimensions before decompensation occurs.

Headache is a common symptom of elevated intracranial pressure and although it may take any form, it is commonly described as deep, steady, and dull. It may be affected by changes in posture and is often worse in the morning. If there is intermittent obstruction of the ventricular system, pain may be sudden and intense. Although the headache is thought to be due to traction on intracranial vessels, its location is not of much value in localizing the position of the intracranial lesion. When headache is severe it is often accompanied by nausea and vomiting. Occasionally, head or neck pain will appear as a result of direct compression or stretching of pain-sensitive cranial or cervical nerves. The appearance of occipital headache in a patient with a supratentorial tumor may point to beginning herniation of the cerebellar tonsils.

Increasing intracranial pressure is transmitted within the prolongations of the arachnoid around the optic nerve. In combination with obstruction to the venous drainage of the eye, it leads to edema of the optic nerve head (papilledema) (Fig. 3.1). Visual acuity is rarely reduced in the early stages of papilledema, but the patient may complain of transient dimness of vision when he stands up quickly. It is essential that the fundi be examined in every patient complaining of headache.

INTRACRANIAL HERNIATIONS

There is evidence that intracranial pressure may be elevated to levels approaching the diastolic blood pressure without serious effects

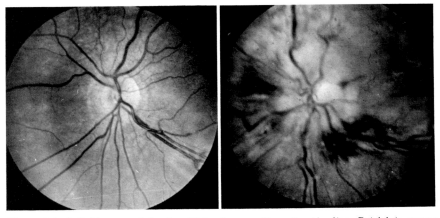

Figure 3.1. A (left): normal fundus. Note sharp outline of optic disc. *B (right):* severe papilledema with marked swelling of optic disc and blurring of its margin. Veins are distended and displaced. There are several fresh hemorrhages into the retina.

so long as the intracranial contents retain their normal anatomic relations. However, if mass and pressure rise in an asymmetric fashion, the soft, almost fluid brain tissue shifts within the skull and herniates through various natural apertures, and serious complications ensue. The direction of the shift and the nature of the herniation will depend upon the location of the expanding mass. The three clinically important shifts are the subfalcine shift of the cerebral midline structures, the transtentorial herniation of the upper brainstem and medial temporal lobes, and herniation of the medulla and cerebellar tonsilar area through the foramen magnum. The term, "pressure cones," is frequently used in relation to the latter two.

Subfalcine Shift

A lesion in one hemisphere, for example a tumor or hematoma, will cause that hemisphere to shift under the falx cerebri to the opposite side. In this fashion, the midline structures below the lower edge of the falx move away from the midline (Fig. 3.2). The lower edge of the falx is at the level of the cingulate gyrus and the latter may become necrotic if severely compressed.

There are no specific neurologic signs produced by this hernia although, occasionally, there may be disturbed function within the territory of the anterior cerebral artery. However, the shift of midline structures is of great clinical importance in that it can be demonstrated by echoencephalography using ultrasound, or by such radiologic techniques as plain skull films (shift of the calcified pineal gland), arteriography (shift of the anterior cerebral artery above the corpus callosum) (Fig. 3.3), and pneumoencephalography (shift and compression of the lateral and third ventricles).

Transtentorial Herniation

This is by far the most important of the herniations. It is a common phenomenon, produces readily recognized clinical manifestations which can be detected at a stage when therapy can be introduced in appropriate circumstances, and is the major direct cause of permanent disability and death from expanding supratentorial masses.

The tentorial aperture is a U-shaped gap formed by the free edge of the tentorium cerebelli and anteriorly by the sphenoid bone. Through it pass the upper brainstem, the posterior cerebral arteries, and the third and sixth cranial nerves (Fig. 3.4), while the medial parts of the temporal lobes (parahippocampal gyri and unci) are related to its lateral edge.

An expanding supratentorial mass will push the posterior diencephalon and medial temporal lobes downward through the aperture into

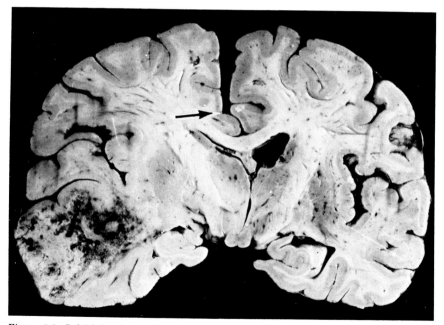

Figure 3.2. Subfalcine herniation due to a tumor in the temporal lobe on the *left*. The third ventricle is shifted about 1.5 cm from the midline position, and it and the lateral ventricle are compressed. There is herniation of the lower part of the cingulate gyrus under the falx cerebri, the lower edge of which was at the *arrow*.

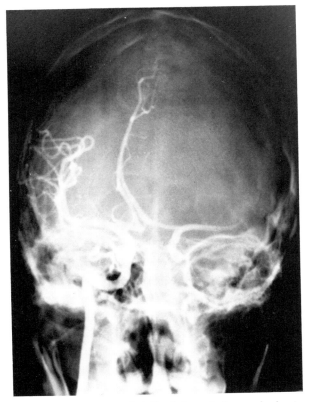

Figure 3.3. Angiogram showing marked shift of the anterior cerebral artery to the *left*, the result of a frontal lobe tumor which has produced a subfalcine herniation.

the posterior fossa (Fig. 3.5). The displacement may be symmetrical, or, if there is a unilateral lesion, it will be more evident on the side of the lesion, with a shift of midline structures away from the lesion.

Among the effects of this herniation are the following:

1. The upper brainstem is compressed and distorted by the displacement (Fig. 3.6). Both venous and arterial blood flow are impaired, leading to hemorrhagic necrosis ("Duret hemorrhages") of the midbrain and upper pons involving particularly the midline and lateral reticular nuclei and the nuclei of the upper cranial nerves. Debate continues regarding the precise mechanics of the distortions and displacement that leads to the vascular lesions.

2. The herniated medial temporal lobes may be compressed and rendered ischemic.

3. The posterior cerebral artery and its calcarine branch are compressed against the edge of the tentorium by the temporal lobe, and hemorrhagic infarction occurs in the medial occipital lobes (Fig. 3.7). Although this in theory would produce unilateral or bilateral homonymous hemianopia, it usually is not apparent clinically because at this stage the patient is comatose and will probably not regain consciousness.

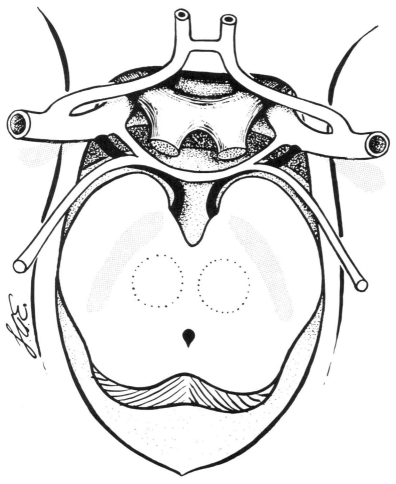

Figure 3.4. Diagram showing relation of structures at the tentorial aperture. Note particularly the course of the third cranial nerves (*black*) under the posterior cerebral arteries, and the relationship of the latter to the free edge of the tentorium.

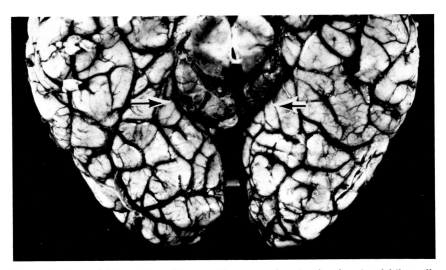

Figure 3.5. Tentorial herniation. The parahippocampal region has herniated bilaterally through the tentorial aperture on both sides of and behind the midbrain (*arrows*). The herniated tissue is congested and hemorrhagic, as is the brainstem, reflecting the local vascular disturbances produced by the hernia.

4. Function of the third nerves is involved, either because the nerves become kinked and stretched in their peripheral course around the posterior cerebral arteries or because their nuclei of origin are involved by the accompanying brainstem lesions.

5. In unilateral lesions, the resulting lateral shift of the upper brainstem may thrust the contralateral cerebral peduncle against the sharp free edge of the tentorium with sufficient force to produce necrosis of the descending fibers (Kernohan's notch) (Fig. 3.8). The resulting pyramidal signs will then be on the same side of the body as the primary cerebral lesion and may thus mislead the clinician.

The compression, distortion, and developing ischemia of the upper brainstem are manifest as impaired consciousness, progressing from drowsiness through stupor to coma. If the original supratentorial lesion is focal in nature, the localizing symptoms and signs arising from that lesion will have grafted upon them the ominous changes in awareness and consciousness pointing to beginning dysfunction in the deep central structures.

With ischemic necrosis and hemorrhage in the upper brainstem, additional signs appear, pointing to the abolition of specific brainstem functions. Eye movements proceed from a stage of divergent roving through a stage when vigorous rotation of the head is necessary to ob-

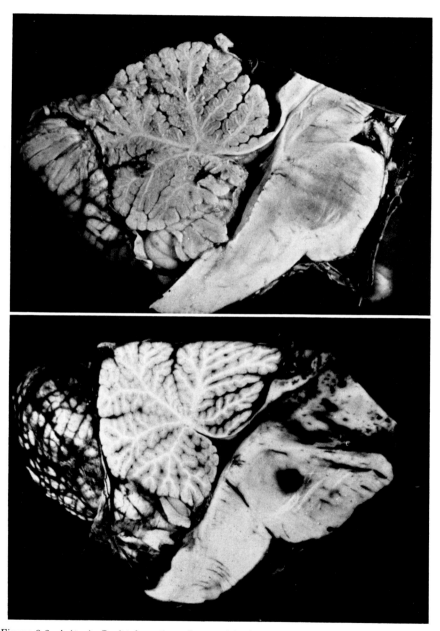

Figure 3.6. A (*top*): Sagittal section of normal brainstem. B (*bottom*): downward compression, distortion, and hemorrhagic necrosis of midbrain and pons produced by tentorial herniation.

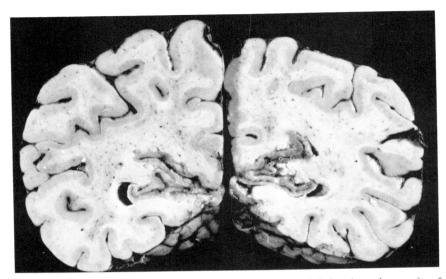

Figure 3.7. Tentorial herniation. Bilateral medial occipital infarction, the result of compression of posterior cerebral arteries at the tentorial aperture.

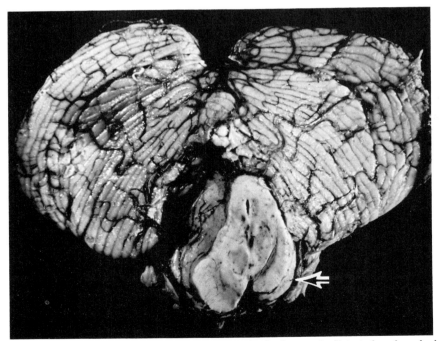

Figure 3.8. Asymmetrical tentorial herniation. The brainstem is distorted and pushed to the *right* of the photograph. The peduncle on this side exhibits necrosis (*arrow*). Note also the midline Duret hemorrhage and compression of the aqueduct.

tain passive movement of the eyes (doll's head movements) to eventual central position and immobility even following caloric stimulation. The latter is performed by irrigating the external auditory canal with cold water. This normally causes the eyes to move conjugately to the opposite side (oculovestibular reflex).

Abnormalities of posture are of important localizing value in the comatose patient. Flexion at the elbows with adduction of the arms across the chest and extension of the legs is known as "decorticate posturing" and implies deep bilateral supratentorial dysfunction. Decerebrate posturing is characterized by stiff extension and adduction of arms and legs with plantar flexion of the feet and points to serious dysfunction at a midbrain level. Release from higher nervous influences in the presence of intact connections between the vestibular nuclei, pontine reticulum, and spinal cord is necessary for the adoption of this posture; it may be elicited in its early stages by applying a painful stimulus to the comatose patient.

Disturbances in breathing may appear and be of Cheyne-Stokes, intermittent, or ataxic types. On rare occasions central neurogenic hyperventilation appears.

The parasympathetic fibers contained in the third cranial nerve and subserving pupillary constriction are affected early. Irritation has been evoked as an explanation for the transient phase of pupillary constriction which may be seen initially. More importantly, however, paralysis of the constrictor muscle leads to dilatation of the pupil with loss of pupillary light reflex. In unilateral lesions, one of the third nerves may be injured before the other, producing a useful lateralizing sign of pupillary inequality, the larger pupil indicating (usually) the side of the lesion.

Pupillary change is often an early and therefore extremely important sign of herniation. Eventually, with advanced herniation, both pupils become dilated and fixed, and external ophthalmoplegia eventually occurs, reflecting further third nerve damage. The retention of pupillary reflexes in a comatose patient suggests a general metabolic or toxic etiology rather than primary intracranial disease.

Some patients may survive the acute period of brainstem compression to be left with variable degrees of neurologic defect, including a state of akinetic mutism or persistent coma with decorticate or decerebrate features. These patients frequently show evidence of necrosis in the midbrain tegmentum and peri-aqueductal region (Fig. 3.9).

Herniation at the Foramen Magnum

Posterior fossa lesions, or diffuse increase in intracranial pressure, have the capacity to force the lower medulla and inferior cerebellum

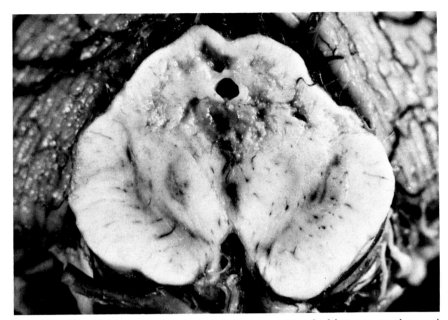

Figure 3.9. Tentorial herniation. A large subdural hematoma had been removed several hours after evidence of brainstem compression occurred. During ensuing month, the patient remained comatose, with fixed, dilated pupils. Death from bronchopneumonia. Note widespread old necrosis with cavitation involving the upper tegmentum and tectum of midbrain.

downward through the foramen magnum (Fig. 3.10). The clinical effects are predominantly those of medullary dysfunction, notably vasomotor collapse and cessation of respiration. Incipient coning may produce discomfort in the occipital area, a stiff neck, or abnormalities in head posture. Extending the neck may produce transient discomfort or short-lived periods of unconsciousness.

Withdrawal of cerebrospinal fluid from the spinal subarachnoid space in the presence of elevated intracranial pressure is a hazardous procedure which may precipitate this herniation and result in the disastrous picture of sudden apnea and loss of consciousness, followed rapidly by death. Lumbar puncture and pneumoencephalography are strongly contraindicated in most patients with clinical evidence of significantly elevated intracranial pressure.

Tumors in the posterior fossa may, on rare occasions, cause upward displacement of the superior cerebellum through the tentorial notch. This may occur suddenly if the supratentorial pressure is lowered by draining the lateral ventricles, or by inserting a hollow needle to carry out the radiologic procedure of ventriculography. This may lead to compression with damage to the dorsal aspect of the midbrain and may obstruct the aqueduct as well as some of the large central veins.

CEREBRAL EDEMA

As with edema elsewhere, cerebral edema has a multitude of precipitating factors, both local and systemic. The mechanisms are as yet poorly understood in many circumstances. The physiologic roles and dynamics of the blood-brain barrier, the blood-cerebrospinal fluid barrier, and the brain-cerebrospinal fluid barrier, and their changes in disease are as yet incompletely known, although much useful experimental and clinical data is available. For the purposes of this monograph, a greatly simplified approach is taken with the assumption that the interested reader will consult the appended references.

The concept of a *blood-brain barrier* was initially based on Ehrlich's observation, in 1885, that certain aniline dyes administered intravenously stained most of the body tissues but did not penetrate the brain. Since then, however, the concept has been greatly expanded to encompass the sum total of the processes, both active and passive,

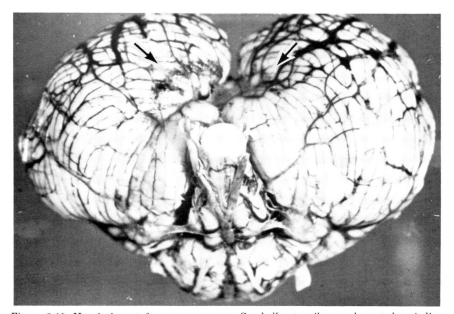

Figure 3.10. Herniation at foramen magnum. Cerebellar tonsils are elongated and displaced downward. Note areas of hemorrhagic necrosis corresponding to compression of cerebellum against posterior edge of foramen magnum (*arrows*).

that serve to regulate the interchange of substances between blood and neural parenchyma. The barrier may prevent, retard, or indeed facilitate passage of individual substances, and thus has the function of carefully regulating the metabolic milieu within the nervous system.

The structural counterparts of the blood-brain barrier include the rather thick non-fenestrated capillary endothelium, the basement membrane, and, surrounding the basement membrane, an essentially continuous sheath formed by the vascular foot processes of astrocytes. Although the evidence is far from complete, the passage of macromolecules such as plasma proteins may be regulated by the endothelium, whereas active electrolyte transport may largely be a function of the glia. The transport of other metabolites such as glucose and amino acids is regulated by a series of active metabolic processes the sites of which are uncertain.

Certain regions in the brain such as the posterior lobe of the pituitary gland, the area postrema, and the pineal body are normally permeable to a number of substances which otherwise are unable to penetrate the brain. This may be related to unusual patterns of vascular anatomy in those regions.

Transfer of substances into the brain or cerebrospinal fluid depends in part upon factors determining transfer across cell membranes in other parts of the body. A substance insoluble in lipid will pass more slowly into brain than one which is lipid-soluble. In general, the larger the molecular size of the substance the slower its penetration.

Monoamines have difficulty entering the central nervous system. In Parkinsonism it has been found that increasing the brain dopamine content results in clinical improvement. However, because dopamine does not penetrate the barrier, its precursor L-DOPA, which can enter the brain, has been given as an oral preparation with resultant symptomatic improvement.

The blood-brain barrier may have other important therapeutic implications by impeding the passage into the central nervous system of drugs such as the antibiotic penicillin. Substances sometimes pass more easily into the brain from the cerebrospinal fluid than from the blood stream and therefore the intrathecal administration of such drugs has been advocated. However, the presence of inflammation of the pia-arachnoid results in increased passage of penicillin leading usually to satisfactory treatment of meningitis by systemic administration alone.

The various functional components of the blood-brain barrier are often altered in disease states. One of the most easily detected alterations is that of increased permeability to substances usually excluded, such as the plasma proteins. An abnormality in electrolyte transport leads to accumulation of sodium in the brain with a concomitant increase in water content. In experimental circumstances a variety of substances are used as tracers to study abnormalities in the various components of blood-brain barrier function.

Cerebral edema is important for two reasons. First, the accumulated fluid produces an increase in cerebral mass and intracranial pressure. Secondly, the edematous tissue fails to function normally and will, in time, undergo degenerative changes which are probably on the basis of fluid stasis and impaired nutrition. A small lesion, for example a metastatic tumor or laceration, may incite a relatively enormous degree of edema and the resulting clinical manifestations are far out of proportion to the size of the primary lesion.

Edema is classified as being local, surrounding a wide variety of focal inflammatory, necrotic, or neoplastic lesions (Fig. 10.14), or generalized, in response to systemic factors or to widespread cerebral damage as occurs in anoxia or heavy metal poisoning (Fig. 3.11).

There are two basic mechanisms operative in the production of cerebral edema. *Vasogenic* edema occurs as the result of increased capillary permeability and is typically seen in the vicinity of focal lesions such as infarcts or tumors. The fluid, which is relatively high in protein, accumulates largely in the extracellular spaces and gradually diffuses through the white matter with some passing through the ependyma into an adjacent ventricular space. The increased content of protein in cerebrospinal fluid found in these lesions is principally due to the presence of such edema fluid.

Cytotoxic edema, in contrast, is an intracellular fluid accumulation resulting from any metabolic disturbance which interferes with the ion pumps controlling cellular hydration. All types of cells may exhibit swelling, but it is best seen in glia and is evident in the early stages in astrocytic perivascular foot processes.

Although relatively pure examples of either type of cerebral edema can be produced in experimental models, one would expect that in most natural diseases they tend to co-exist, either sequentially or simultaneously. In human pathology, most examples of significant edema appear to have a major vasogenic component.

Edematous brain tissue appears swollen, somewhat softened, and translucent. White matter is more prone to swelling than gray, although compact fiber tracts are relatively resistant. In longstanding edema, the tissue becomes yellowish and quite soft, and may eventually become cystic. Histologically, tissue elements appear separated by accumulated fluid; myelin sheaths, and later axons, become irregular, beaded, and vacuolated, and they eventually break down. In chronic edema there is

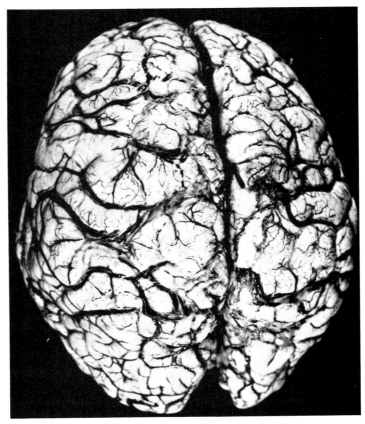

Figure 3.11. Cerebral edema, generalized, following cardiac arrest. The brain weight was about 150 g more than normal; on the external surface the sulci appear compressed and gyri are flattened as a result of compression against the inside of the skull. There is also venous congestion.

widespread astrocytic hyperplasia and hypertrophy which, in a small cerebral biopsy, may resemble a low-grade astrocytic tumor and lead to diagnostic error.

The important diagnostic procedure of radioisotope scanning (Fig. 10. 10) is based on the increased permeability of vessels within and adjacent to focal lesions. A gamma emitter which does not pass the normal blood-brain barrier to any extent, but which accumulates in the abnormally permeable region, is given intravenously and a scan of the calvaria is performed a few minutes or hours later. Although the procedure is generally used for the localization of tumors, it must be remembered that any destructive lesion may give a positive result.

Since cerebral edema may be a life-threatening complication of an otherwise self-limited or remediable lesion, its control is of obvious therapeutic importance. Large volumes of hypertonic solutions such as urea, mannitol, or sucrose, administered intravenously, will reduce swelling by their osmotic effect, although the effect is short-lived as the blood returns to isotonicity. Large doses of corticosteroids are sometimes effective in reducing edema and are often used to lessen traumatic edema and following surgical manipulation of the brain.

Benign Intracranial Hypertension

This is a relatively uncommon disorder of considerable theoretical interest which may present the clinician with a difficult problem in investigation and management. It most frequently affects young women, particularly those who are somewhat overweight, and there is often a history of menstrual irregularity.

The clinical manifestations are those of elevated intracranial pressure—headache, nausea and vomiting, and papilledema—without localizing signs, although diplopia may appear due to unilateral or bilateral third or sixth nerve palsy. Pneumoencephalography occasionally shows the ventricles to be compressed, suggesting cerebral edema, although they may be of normal size. The cerebrospinal fluid pressure may be elevated to between 300 and 600 mm of water. The cause is unknown, although disordered endocrine function is postulated by some. The condition is usually self-limited over a period of a few months. In a few cases, the papilledema may result in optic atrophy and residual visual impairment, and surgical decompression may be required to preserve vision.

A similar syndrome may occur in hypoparathyroidism, vitamin A toxicity, hypoadrenalism, long-term adrenal corticosteroid therapy, and with tetracycline administration. In these latter conditions the pathogenesis is obscure.

HYDROCEPHALUS

Hydrocephalus is the accumulation within the cranial cavity of an excessive amount of cerebrospinal fluid. Hydrocephalus *ex vacuo* is simply the increase in fluid occurring when the brain has become atrophic and no longer fills the cranial cavity.

True hydrocephalus may occur on the basis of one of three mechanisms.

1. Most cases of hydrocephalus are due to obstruction to the flow of cerebrospinal fluid (obstructive hydrocephalus).

2. The resorptive capacity may be reduced by fibrosis of the arachnoid granulations or by extensive thrombosis of the dural venous sinuses. The latter, formerly seen as a complication of infection, is now uncommon.

3. The excretion of cerebrospinal fluid may be excessive, exceeding the resorptive capacity. This may occur as a feature of papillomas of the choroid plexus (Fig. 3.12), but its existence is doubted by many.

Obstructive hydrocephalus occurs as the result of a lesion which interferes with the circulation of cerebrospinal fluid from the choroid plexuses to the arachnoid granulations, at any point along the pathways. The lesion may be congenital—for example, atresia of the aqueduct of Sylvius (Fig. 3.13) or of the foramina of Luschka or Magendie, or the Arnold-Chiari malformation (Fig. 3.14). Among the many acquired lesions that may be responsible, the most important are meningeal fibrosis following infection and hemorrhage (Fig. 3.15) and critically located tumors in the area of the aqueduct or third or fourth ventricles (Fig. 10.8).

The site of obstruction determines which of the ventricles will be

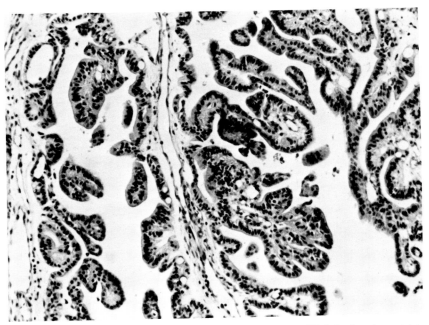

Figure 3.12. Choroid plexus papilloma. A papillary tumor mass filled the fourth ventricle, producing hydrocephalus, most likely on an obstructive basis. The histologic features of the tumor have a resemblance to the normal choroid plexus. (Hematoxylin-eosin, × 400)

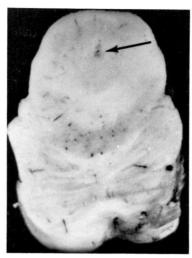

Figure 3.13. Aqueduct stenosis. The lumen of aqueduct was of microscopic dimensions and is not seen in the photograph. The surrounding area, (*arrow*) which appears gray and somewhat translucent, is composed of glial tissue.

affected. If the obstruction is in the basal meninges, the entire ventricular system is dilated, while an obstruction within the ventricular system produces dilatation proximal to the site.

The pathologic effects are in part age-dependent. Before the cranial sutures have closed in the fetus or infant, the accumulated fluid causes the entire cranium to expand, sometimes to balloon-like proportions (Fig. 3.16). Within the very thin skull, only a paper-thin remnant of the cortical mantle may persist (Fig. 3.17). Serial measurements of the diameter of the infant head are an important component of the physical examination, permitting early recognition of abnormal enlargement at a stage when treatment is still of benefit. The rate of growth of the head over a period of observation is more important than the head size at any one time. With advanced hydrocephalus, there appear mental retardation, a characteristic downward displacement of eyes, and papilledema which may proceed to optic atrophy. Involvement of the corticospinal tracts, especially the leg fibers which have a longer intracranial course, leads to spastic paraplegia. Air studies are of importance in determining the location of the obstruction and the severity of cerebral atrophy (Fig. 3.18).

In older children and adults, the skull is incapable of expansion and therefore the obstruction produces an elevation of intracranial pressure, with subsequent ventricular dilatation, and brain atrophy chiefly of

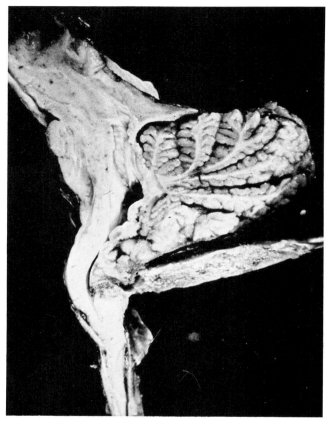

Figure 3.14. Arnold-Chiari malformation. This is a complex malformation of structures forming and contained within the posterior fossa. The brainstem is hypoplastic and markedly elongated, so that the fourth ventricle extends into the upper cervical canal. A tongue of cerebellar vermis also extends through the foramen magnum, and the foramen of Magendie is obstructed. Note the "beaking" of the tectal plate of the midbrain. The aqueduct of Sylvius, not visible in the photograph, was atretic, and the lateral and third ventricles were enormously dilated.

white matter. The cortex and basal ganglia may be quite well-preserved, and intellect and behavior may often be surprisingly well-maintained in the presence of considerable ventricular enlargement. It is difficult to predict the clinical findings from looking at the size of the ventricles, but, as a general rule, the greatest disturbance in mental functions will be seen in patients with the most pronounced degree of cerebral atrophy.

The mechanisms of cerebral atrophy in obstructive hydrocephalus are of some current interest. The ependymal lining, which normally has an active metabolic role in brain-cerebrospinal fluid interchange, stretches and finally breaks to permit free interchange of cerebral intersitial fluid and cerebrospinal fluid, and this probably has a deleterious effect on the metabolism of white matter near the ventricles. As the ventricles enlarge, their surface area increases. The force (pressure × area) exerted on adjacent structures is thus increased as well. It has been proposed that as the ventricles dilate, a lower pressure is able to provide the force required to produce continuing periventricular damage. In some instances, notably in older adults, the pressure is only slightly elevated or near the upper limit of the normal range (normal pressure hydrocephalus), but in spite of this there is increasing disability. In such patients, clinical improvement may follow surgical procedures designed to reduce intracranial pressure.

The treatment of hydrocephalus is based on surgically establishing artificial channels (shunts) for drainage of cerebrospinal fluid in order to keep the intraventricular pressure within physiologic limits. To be useful, this must of course be undertaken before significant cerebral atrophy has developed; there is little benefit in maintaining life after cortical function is lost. Commonly used shunts are plastic tubes with various types of pumps and valves, one end inserted into a ventricle and

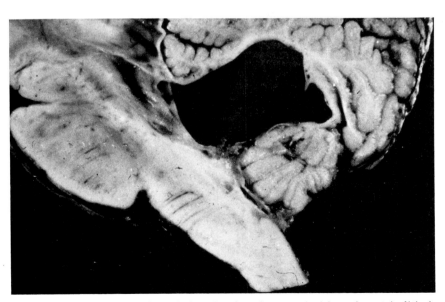

Figure 3.15. Obstructive hydrocephalus. Purulent leptomeningitis and ventriculitis in infancy resulted in extensive fibrosis which occluded the outlet foramina of the fourth ventricle and produced hydrocephalus.

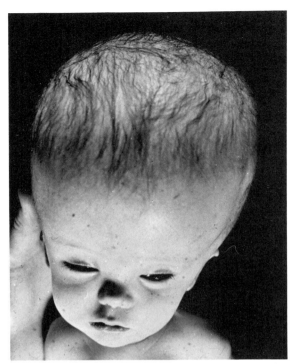

Figure 3.16. Infantile hydrocephalus due to aqueductal stenosis. The calvaria is markedly enlarged in a symmetrical fashion, making the face seem small by comparison.

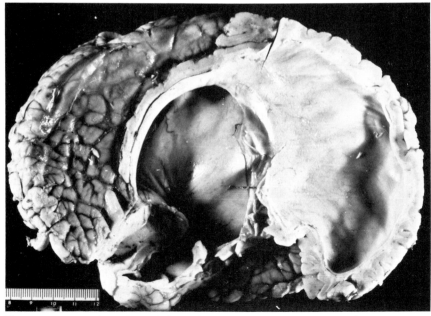

Figure 3.17. Infantile hydrocephalus. The brain is markedly enlarged due to enormous dilatation of the lateral ventricles. Only a thin rim of cortex and adjacent white matter persists.

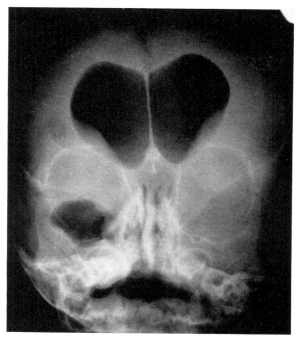

Figure 3.18. Pneumoencephalogram. Hydrocephalus due to aqueduct stenosis in a 5 month old boy. Note the gross symmetrical enlargement of lateral ventricles, including the one temporal horn containing air.

the other into the pleural or peritoneal cavities or the right atrium of the heart.

EXAMINATION OF THE CEREBROSPINAL FLUID

Cerebrospinal fluid examination is indicated whenever it can be expected to assist clinical diagnosis. The fluid is withdrawn by inserting a needle, under aseptic techniques, into the lumbar subarachnoid sac below the lower end of the spinal cord at the Lumbar 3-4 or 4-5 interspace. Fluid may also be obtained by lateral ventricular tap and from the cisterna magna, but these procedures are hazardous in inexperienced hands.

There are two major contraindications to lumbar puncture. When intracranial pressure is elevated, there is a risk of producing a cerebellomedullary pressure cone and death. However, if pressure is judged clinically to be only mildly elevated and the diagnostic or therapeutic benefits expected of the examination are great, the risk may be justified.

If the tissues through which the needle is to pass are infected, there is a considerable risk of producing meningitis.

Analysis of the cellular, chemical, and microbiologic elements of cerebrospinal fluid is of considerable assistance in diagnosis or exclusion of specific diseases. If one has a clear idea of the mechanism of the various changes, their significance becomes readily apparent.

Appearance

Cerebrospinal fluid is a clear, colorless watery fluid. A red color is imparted by blood; a yellow color (xanthochromia) indicates breakdown products of hemoglobin or, less often, a very high protein content. Turbidity is produced by a high leukocytic content or by coagulation of a fibrin skein.

Pressure

Pressure is measured clinically using a manometer attached to the needle. The normal pressure in a person lying on his side and reasonably relaxed is about 60 to 180 mm of cerebrospinal fluid (4 to 14 mm of mercury). Small oscillations occur with respiration and pulse, and large elevations are produced by coughing or jugular venous compression. Blockage of the spinal arachnoid space may abolish the latter (Queckenstedt's test).

More accurate measurements of pressure and of dynamic changes are made with appropriate transducers and recording apparatus which avoid the considerable damping effect of the needle and manometer. Indwelling ventricular catheters may be used to monitor continuously intracranial pressure in situations when it may fluctuate, such as following head injuries.

Cellular Elements

Erythrocytes and leukocytes are identified and counted using techniques similar to those in hematology with dilutions appropriate to the much lower cell count.

Erythrocytes, normally absent from cerebrospinal fluid, appear as the result of any bleeding into the subarachnoid space following primary hemorrhage, tissue necrosis, or trauma. They may also be derived from a "traumatic" lumbar puncture with damage to local blood vessels.

Grossly bloody fluid may be centrifuged. A clear supernatant indicates that the red cells have been there for a very short time, whereas xanthochromia indicates that there has been sufficient time (at least

3 to 4 hours) for some lysis to occur. Bleeding from a traumatic tap usually stops in a few minutes, and a second or third tube of fluid taken after a short interval will thus contain fewer erythrocytes.

Normal cerebrospinal fluid may contain as many as five leukocytes per ml, all mononuclear cells (lymphocytes and macrophages); a count of 10 or more white cells is indicative of a disease process.

Recent bleeding will, of course, contribute circulating leukocytes; a calculation of the number derived from this source can be made by counting both leukocytes and erythrocytes and relating these figures to counts made on the circulating blood.

Neutrophils in cerebrospinal fluid are always to be regarded as abnormal. Large numbers (in excess of 100) are highly suggestive of infection by pyogenic bacteria, and lower counts are present in other infections and following recent necrosis.

Mononuclear cells are also evidence of an inflammatory process, particularly in the lower-grade bacterial and fungal infections, viral diseases, and some destructive processes such as disseminated sclerosis.

Lesions involving a meningeal surface generally produce higher cell counts than equivalent deeper ones; for example, in a deep-seated cerebral abscess, very few leukocytes may find their way into cerebrospinal fluid.

Slowly progressive degenerative diseases are not usually associated with increased cell counts.

Cytologic examination of cerebrospinal fluid for malignant cells may be useful when tumor has invaded the meninges and particularly in the detection of meningeal carcinomatoses.

Chemical Constituents

Protein

The selective mechanisms involved in cerebrospinal fluid formation are effective in almost eliminating protein; the normal level is less than 45 mg per 100 ml. Fifty to 70 percent of the protein is albumin and the rest is globulin. Fibrinogen is absent. The electrophoretic pattern is similar to that of serum. Ventricular fluid protein is considerably lower, below 20 mg per 100 ml.

Elevation of protein is the commonest abnormality of cerebrospinal fluid and is always indicative of a pathologic process. A level of 50 mg per 100 ml or more, reported from a carefully monitored laboratory, always requires investigation. However, a normal level by no means excludes chronic neurologic disease.

The principal sources of elevated protein are lesions that alter vascular permeability in brain or meninges, permitting the escape of plasma proteins. As with other exudates, albumin escapes in relatively greater amounts than other proteins. The presence of fibrinogen indicates massive change in permeability, and occurs occasionally in tuberculosis and other infections.

Occasionally, as in multiple sclerosis and neurosyphilis, gamma-globulin may be disproportionately elevated (greater than 20 percent of the total protein) in the presence of normal or only slightly elevated total protein. There is some evidence that in these circumstances the excess globulin is not derived from plasma but is formed locally by lymphoid and plasma cells in the inflammatory exudate associated with the lesions.

Glucose

The cerebrospinal fluid glucose value is about 20 to 30 mg per 100 ml below the blood level, and rises and falls with the latter after a lag of about 2 hours. An elevated level is of no significance except that it reflects hyperglycemia.

A reduced level, below 40 mg per 100 ml, is characteristic of bacterial and fungal meningitis, meningeal sarcoidosis, and widespread tumor involvement of meninges. In these circumstances, it is postulated that the abnormal cells and organisms metabolize the glucose, and there may also be interference in active transport of glucose from the blood stream.

Other Substances

Electrolytes, ammonia, amino acids, lipids, enzymes, and a wide variety of other substances in cerebrospinal fluid have been measured in health and disease states, but have limited diagnostic application.

Microbiologic Examination

In infectious diseases, the causative organisms may be found in direct smears or cultures, or by animal inoculation, and the antibiotic sensitivities may be determined where applicable. In some infections, specific antibodies in cerebrospinal fluid may be of diagnostic significance. It is of importance to emphasize that failure to identify organisms by no means rules out the presence of an infection; occasionally, repeated attempts must be made.

REFERENCES

BAKAY, L., AND LEE, J. C. Cerebral Edema. Charles C Thomas, Publisher, Inc., Springfield, Ill., 1965.

CROME, L., AND STERN, J. The Pathology of Mental Retardation. Little, Brown & Co., Boston, 1967.

DAVSON, H. Physiology of the Cerebrospinal Fluid. Little, Brown & Co., Boston, 1967.

FISHMAN, R. A. Cerebrospinal fluid. *In* Clinical Neurology, Vol. 1. Ed. by A. B. Baker. Hoeber Medical Division, Harper and Row, Publishers, New York, 1962.

HILL, M. E., LOUGHEED, W. M., AND BARNETT, H. J. M. A treatable form of dementia due to normal-pressure, communicating hydrocephalus. Canad. Med. Ass. J. 97:1309, 1967.

KLATZO, I. Neuropathological aspects of brain edema. J. Neuropath. Exp. Neurol. 26:1, 1967.

KLATZO, I., AND SEITELBERGER, F. (Eds). Brain Edema. Springer-Verlag, New York, 1967.

KLINTWORTH, G. K. The pathogenesis of secondary brainstem hemorrhages as studied in an experimental model. Amer. J. Path. 47:525, 1965.

RUSSELL, D. S. Observations on the Pathology of Hydrocephalus. Medical Research Council No. 265. Her Majesty's Stationery Office, London, 1949.

TOWBIN, A. Central nervous system damage in the human fetus and newborn infant. Amer. J. Dis. Child. 119:529, 1970.

4

METABOLIC AND NUTRITIONAL DISORDERS

INTRODUCTION

An increasing number of circumstances are recognized in which disordered cerebral function and structure occur as the result of systemic metabolic disturbances. The sensitivity to changes in their metabolic milieu of individual neurons and to a lesser extent of neuroglia was discussed in Chapter 2. Some examples of the way disturbed metabolism and nutrition affect the nervous system will be examined in this chapter. Much work remains to be done in investigating this field although there have been significant advances in recent years.

For purposes of discussion, the metabolic disorders may be divided as follows: (1) inborn metabolic errors affecting the nervous system; (2) anoxia and hypoglycemia; (3) deficiency diseases; (4) neurologic disturbances secondary to hepatic, renal, endocrine, and other systemic disease.

INBORN ERRORS OF METABOLISM

The essential and genetically determined factor in an inborn error of metabolism is the absence or inactivity of one or more enzymes. In some diseases, the specific enzyme defect is known. With others, much is known about the nature of the disturbed metabolism, but the definitive enzymatic defect has not yet been identified. These disorders usually have a recessive pattern of inheritance and occasionally arise as mutations. Heterozygotes may show a partial deficiency of an enzyme but are usually able to function well under normal circumstances, whereas homozygotes will show absence of the enzyme and the presence of clinical disease.

Among the numerous inborn metabolic errors now identified, many are associated with mental retardation, motor disturbances, blindness, deafness, peripheral neuropathy, or other evidence of neurologic disease. Among the numerous familial neurologic diseases in which a meta-bolic defect has not been demonstrated, some will undoubtedly prove to be inborn metabolic errors, although with others, environmental or other non-genetic factors may be responsible.

The major categories of inherited disease arising from a disorder of metabolism and affecting the nervous system are those with disturb-ances in metabolism of amino acids, sphingolipid, carbohydrate, or mucopolysaccharide. Characteristic examples will be taken from the first two groups.

Inborn Errors of Amino Acid Metabolism

Systematic study of large populations of mentally retarded children has led to the discovery of some of the aminoacidurias as well as other diseases arising on the basis of enzyme defects. However, it must be emphasized that a metabolic defect is found in only a small minority of defective children. Most cases of severe mental deficiency are the re-sult of cerebral malformations, birth injuries, or infections.

Phenylketonuria, the commonest aminoaciduria, is diagnosed by the finding of hyperphenylalaninemia due to the absence of the enzyme, phenylalanine hydroxylase, blocking the pathway for the breakdown of phenylalanine. The most frequent finding is mental retardation; how-ever, the effects on the brain of deletion (or inactivity) of the enzyme are to some extent unpredictable and the mechanism is not fully under-stood. A small minority of individuals are of normal intelligence and the remainder show a wide range of mental ability extending from border-line intelligence to idiocy.

There is little evidence that phenylalanine or its metabolities are di-rectly toxic to neurons or glia at concentrations found in phenylketo-nuria. A secondary effect on tryptophan and 5-hydroxytryptamine metabolism may be more directly related to the cerebral dysfunction.

The morphologic changes in the brain in the aminoacidurias vary widely but are often minimal and appear insignificant in comparison to the magnitude of the clinical defect. In some, the weight of the brain is less than normal (microcephaly) and cortical neurons appear reduced in number or are smaller and less well-developed than expected for the patient's age. In others, hypomyelination or breakdown of myelin is found. However, the minor morphologic changes found in many of these patients may be due to nutritional disturbances or intercurrent disease rather than to the primary metabolic defect.

There is considerable evidence that a phenylalanine-free diet insti-tuted in infancy will lessen the degree of cerebral damage, but debate continues as to the likelihood of normal intellectual development in these circumstances. It has not been possible to replace the enzyme phenylalanine hydroxylase.

Inborn Errors of Sphingolipid Metabolism

It has been known for some time that in several inherited neurologic diseases, loss of neurons, myelin sheaths, or both is associated with the accumulation of complex sphingolipids in neural tissues, with involvement of other organs as well in some instances. Historically, several classifications have been based on clinical or pathologic findings but in the past few years rapid progress in this field has rendered obsolete much of the old terminology.

In the sphingolipidoses in which the enzyme defect is known, a lysosomal hydrolase involved in sphingolipid catabolism is absent or exhibits attenuated activity, and, as a result, a specific lipid accumulates in the tissues. Some examples are briefly outlined here.

Ganglioside Storage Diseases

Most of the gangliosides in the nervous system are contained in neurons where they presumably play a role in cell membrane and synaptic transmission. A deficiency in any one of the several enzymes responsible for their step-wise degradation results in the accumulation of a ganglioside, predominantly in neurons, but to a lesser extent in glia and macrophages. This group of diseases (there are at least five) are collectively known as the cerebral lipidoses or ganglioside storage diseases.

The most common is Tay-Sach's disease, in which ganglioside GM2 accumulates as a result of deficiency of a hexosamidase A. In this disease, the defective gene is almost confined to descendants of Ashkenazi Jews. The affected infant usually appears normal at birth, but by 3 to 6 months demonstrates evidence of mental and motor deterioration, followed by progressive blindness, deafness, paralysis, and finally a state of decerebrate rigidity. Death usually occurs by the age of 4 years. The head is frequently enlarged in the early stages as the result of the lipid accumulation. Neurons are massively distended by lipid (Fig. 4.1) which is contained within small membrane-bound intracytoplasmic bodies derived from lysosomes. Lipid also accumulates in autonomic nerve cells so that a rectal biopsy may be of assistance in diagnosis by revealing lipid-laden ganglion cells in Meissner's plexus. Retinal ganglion cell involvement renders the retina opaque and gray-white in color. The macula, which is devoid of ganglion cells, remains transparent and

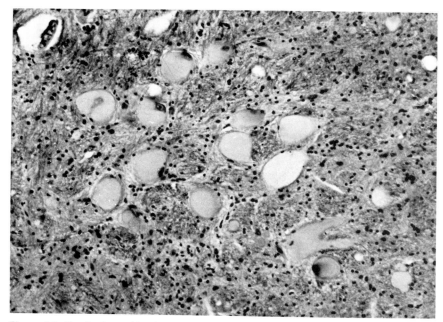

Figure 4.1. Cerebral gangliosidosis GM2 (Tay-Sach's disease). Neurons of the motor nucleus of the fifth cranial nerve are massively distended by the accumulated ganglioside, and nuclei are displaced to the margins. Contrast with normal motor neuron in Figure 2.10*A*. (Luxol fast blue-hematoxylin-eosin (LFB-HE), × 130)

appears as a "cherry-red spot," a striking clinical feature present in most cases.

The other ganglioside storage diseases are similar but differ in their specific biochemical features, age of onset, rate of progression, and presence or absence of lipid (or mucopolysaccharide) storage in the liver, kidneys, spleen, and other viscera.

Cerebroside Storage Diseases

Galactocerebroside and cerebroside sulfate are important constituents of myelin. Deficiency of their specific hydrolytic enzymes produces myelin breakdown and accumulation of the cerebroside in white matter both within macrophages (Fig. 4.2) and apparently free in the extracellular spaces. Secondary axonal loss and gliosis also occur. Damage is diffuse, involving both peripheral and central myelinated fibers in all areas. On gross examination, atrophy, gliosis, and discolora-

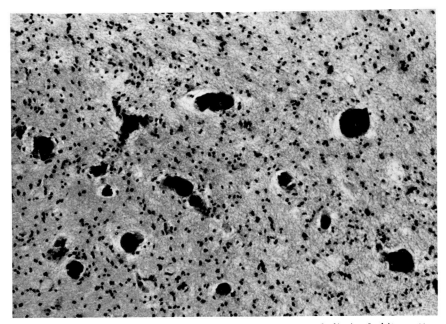

Figure 4.2. Krabbe's disease. There is marked loss of myelin and gliosis of white matter, and clusters of macrophages distended with cerebroside ("globoid cells") are scattered throughout. (Hematoxylin-eosin (HE), × 130)

tion are most evident in large myelinated areas such as the centrum semiovale (Fig. 4.3).

The term "leukodystrophy" is applied to those genetically based diseases in which white matter lesions predominate, and includes galactocerebroside storage (Krabbe's disease) and cerebroside sulfate storage (metachromatic leukodystrophy). In contrast, in glucocerebroside storage (Gaucher's disease), the accumulations are predominantly in liver, bone marrow, spleen, and reticuloendothelial system. In brain, little glucocerebroside is present and therefore resultant pathologic accumulation is also usually slight.

There are other leukodystrophies in which the metabolic defect is not evident, or in which no abnormal accumulation of lipid has been demonstrated.

Diagnosis of Sphingolipidoses

The clinical features in this group of diseases are rarely distinctive enough to permit accurate diagnosis. Before the enzyme deficiencies were recognized, resort was made to biopsy of such tissues as peripheral nerve, rectal myenteric plexus, brain, liver, and bone marrow, with subsequent histochemical and chemical characterization of the stored lipid. Now, however, in most instances specific enzyme assays may be performed on white cells, serum, urine, or cultured skin fibroblasts. Carriers can be identified in some of the diseases.

Recently, it has been shown that these and other inborn metabolic errors can be demonstrated before birth by assays performed on cultures of aspirated amniotic cells. Parents carrying a known genetic defect may thus decide whether they wish pregnancy interrupted, based on a clear indication of whether or not the fetus has acquired the disorder.

ANOXIA AND HYPOGLYCEMIA

Anoxia, hypoglycemia, and generalized cerebral ischemia of systemic origin (for example, during cardiac arrest) have similar effects upon the brain.

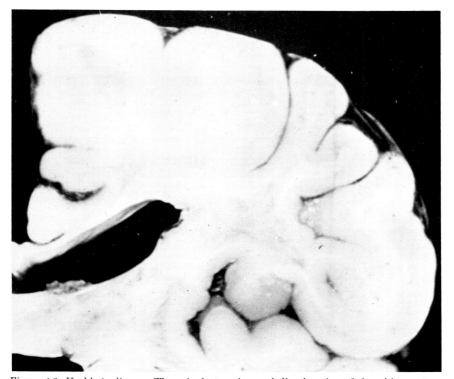

Figure 4.3. Krabbe's disease. There is destruction and discoloration of the white matter of the centrum semiovale and marked thinning of the corpus callosum. The cerebral cortex and the subcortical "U" fibers are relatively spared.

If cerebral circulation is completely and abruptly stopped, unconsciousness occurs within 10 to 15 seconds, reflecting the remarkable dependency of neurons on a continuous supply of oxygen and glucose. Within 5 to 10 minutes, the most susceptible neurons die, notably in cerebral cortex (particularly the third layer of pyramidal cells and the hippocampus), cerebellar cortex, and globus pallidus. Most nuclei in the diencephalon, brainstem, and spinal cord are considerably more resistant and may survive for as long as 30 or more minutes. If circulation is restored after several minutes of cardiac arrest, brain function may be retained in the form of continuation of lower functions, but the loss of cortical neurons results in dementia with signs of focal or generalized cerebral damage.

Hypoglycemia may appear with insulin-secreting tumors or liver disease or may be induced by insulin overdose. Hypoglycemia is associated clinically with autonomic effects such as sweating and tachycardia due to release of large amounts of epinephrine and central effects due to the removal of the main metabolic substrate of the brain. Drowsiness, confusion, and delirium appear as blood glucose levels drop to 30 mg per 100 ml, and coma, often with seizures, occurs at about 20 mg per 100 ml. Lower levels result in neuronal loss which has a similar distribution to that of anoxia. Recently, infantile hypoglycemia has been recognized as a significant cause of neonatal brain damage.

Poisoning with carbon monoxide, barbiturates, or cyanide, respiratory obstruction, intra-uterine and perinatal anoxia, and other types of acute anoxia produce similar lesions. Minor differences in the distribution of lesions are described, but in all cases, the predominant clinical effects reflect the particular sensitivity of the cortical neurons.

The cortical lesions in anoxia and hypoglycemia consist of widespread neuronal loss and later gliosis, involving all layers but particularly the third (Fig. 4.4). There is a tendency for lesions to be most severe in the boundry zones between the cerebral arteries and in the depths of sulci where blood flow may be somewhat less. The band-like cortical lesions are referred to as "pseudolaminar necrosis." Purkinje cells are destroyed in the cerebellum, whereas the more resistant granule cells are usually preserved. The brain is diffusely edematous in the acute phase, and there may be evidence of myelin vacuolation and fragmentation. In survivors, there is occasionally widespread patchy demylination and gliosis of white matter, possibly the result of edema or oligodendroglial necrosis. An unexplained phenomenon is the occasional finding of severe white matter lesions in the face of minimal loss of cortical neurons.

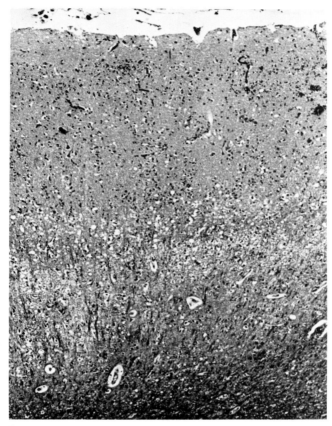

Figure 4.4. Pseudolaminar necrosis of cerebral cortex. Severe hypoglycemia of unknown duration following an overdose of insulin. Necrosis in this field is maximal in the deeper layers. (LFB-HE, × 40)

DEFICIENCY DISEASES

It is well recognized that poorly nourished children of impoverished families often fail to achieve normal intellectual development. Many factors are involved, including genetic and environmental influences and educational opportunities. Maternal malnutrition may have a detrimental effect on fetal development. It is also apparent that a diet suboptimal in caloric content, protein, or other essential factors has a detrimental effect on the growth and maturation of the brain. The critical period appears to be infancy and early childhood at which time the brain undergoes most of its growth.

Specific nutritional deficiency diseases present many interesting problems to the investigator. In most instances, a knowledge of intermediary metabolism suggests a number of mechanisms by which a specific deficiency could be harmful. These diseases tend to affect specific areas of the nervous system, presumably the result of as yet undisclosed metabolic peculiarities of cells in these areas. Some deficiencies predominantly affect neurons whereas others involve glia. Examples of this group of diseases are those disorders arising from deficiencies of the B group of vitamins.

The B vitamins involved in carbohydrate metabolism are essential to nervous function. Deficiencies of thiamine, riboflavin, and niacin result in degeneration of peripheral axons and their myelin sheaths, producing the clinical picture of distal polyneuropathy (nutritional polyneuropathy) with sensory and motor impairment and loss of reflexes (Fig. 4.5). An additional effect of severe thiamine deficiency, most often seen

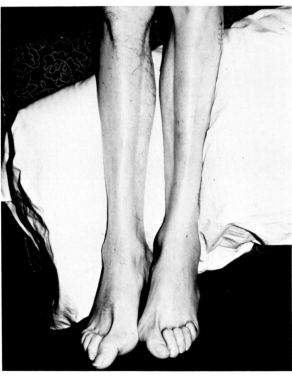

Figure 4.5. Nutritional polyneuropathy. Chronic alcoholic. Moderate wasting of leg muscles. There was weakness, particularly of dorsiflexion, impairment of all sensory modalities, and ankle areflexia.

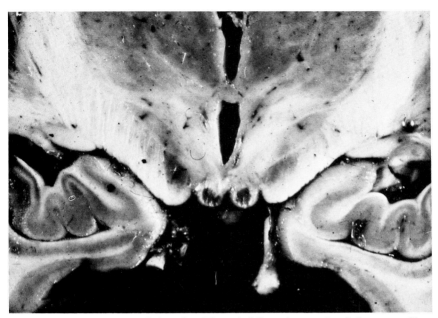

Figure 4.6. Wernicke's encephalopathy. There is bilateral necrosis of the mammillary bodies and of the adjacent hypothalamus near the third ventricle.

in chronic alcoholics, is Wernicke's encephalopathy. There is selective damage of the posterior hypothalamus including the mamillary bodies (Fig. 4.6), portions of the tegmentum of the upper brainstem, and vestibular nuclei. The clinical picture includes drowsiness, disturbed mentation, extra-ocular paralysis, and nystagmus. Early signs result from still reversible neuronal dysfunction with localized edema of the involved areas. At this stage, administration of thiamine produces a prompt and dramatic clinical response. However, if the diagnosis is overlooked and the patient remains untreated, neuronal necrosis and hemorrhage supervene and if the patient lives he is left with permanent impairment of new learning and recent memory for which he may compensate by confabulation (Korsakoff's psychosis). The fully developed syndrome is not responsive to therapy with thiamine.

Occasionally, chronic alcoholics develop a slowly progressive cerebellar syndrome with ataxia of legs and trunk predominating. Pathologically there is cerebellar atrophy, largely confined to the superior vermis and adjacent superior surfaces of the hemispheres (Fig. 4.7), which histologically exhibits loss of Purkinje cells and, to a lesser degree, of granule cells (Fig. 4.8). The cause is unknown, although in most cases there is associated evidence of multiple nutritional deficiencies.

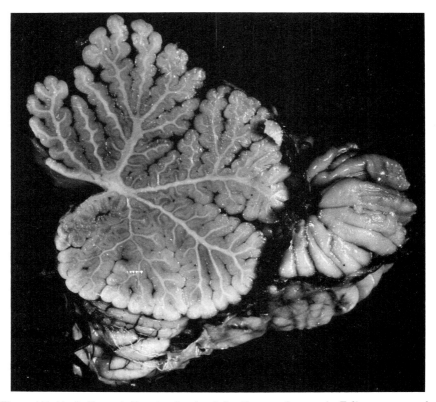

Figure 4.7. Alcoholic cerebellar atrophy, involving the superior vermis. Folia are narrowed and sulci are widened.

In pernicious anemia and in other forms of vitamin B12 deficiency, the syndrome of subacute combined degeneration may occur, usually but not invariably in association with characteristic hematologic findings. Degeneration of the lateral and dorsal long tracts of the spinal cord is present and most pronounced in the midthoracic region, with vacuolation and degeneration of myelin sheaths and axonal loss, accompanied by remarkably little astrocytic response (Fig. 4.9). Patchy focal demyelination often occurs in the cerebral hemispheres, and there is a peripheral neuropathy. Patients therefore may present with evidence of disturbed mental function, spinal cord damage, or peripheral sensory and motor findings. The metabolic defect presumably affects oligodendroglia and the failure of gliosis may also indicate a glial abnormality. After therapy, the involved spinal areas undergo intense gliosis. Signs of spinal cord damage respond less well to treatment than those of peripheral nerve involvement.

It will be apparent that early and accurate diagnosis of deficiency diseases of the nervous system is essential so that adequate replacement therapy can be started before irreparable damage has occurred.

NEUROLOGIC DISORDERS SECONDARY TO HEPATIC, RENAL, ENDOCRINE, AND OTHER SYSTEMIC DISORDERS

Previous sections of this chapter outline the way in which the nervous system suffers from the effects of systemic anoxia and hypoglycemia due to a diminished supply of oxygen, metabolic substrate, or cofactors. Metabolic encephalopathies can also develop in association with diseases of the liver, kidney, thyroid, and other organs. Additional causes include respiratory disease with hypoventilation, poisoning by drugs, both hypo-osmolar and hyperosmolar states, and hypocalcemia as may occur with hypoparathyroidism. It is therefore obvious that the clinician must be aware of the many intrinsic, extrinsic, and toxic conditions which can produce disturbed mentation leading eventually to

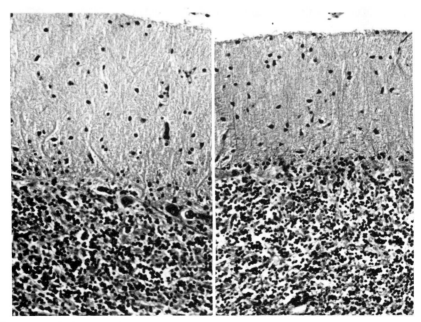

Figure 4.8. Alcoholic cerebellar atrophy. *A* (*left*): inferior vermis, essentially uninvolved. *B* (*right*): superior vermis, with marked thinning of molecular layer and loss of Purkinje cells. (*A* and *B*, LFB-HE, × 100)

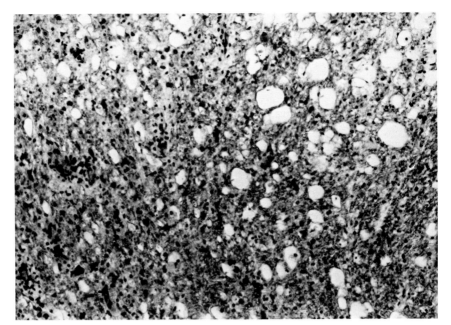

Figure 4.9. Subacute combined degeneration. Lateral column of thoracic cord. Marked reticulation and myelin loss and infiltration by macrophages. (Loyez, × 120)

coma. Patients may show similar symptoms no matter which systemic disorder is responsible. The patient may pass through a period of apathy and drowsiness, inattentiveness, and disturbances in memory. Tremor and sudden lapses of posture of the arms may appear, occasionally punctuated by myoclonic movements or seizures. Frequently, these mental and motor disturbances show considerable fluctuation in severity in the early stages. As the metabolic condition worsens, consciousness steadily declines, proceeding to coma.

When a patient arrives at the emergency department in coma it is necessary not only to carry out such immediate measures as ensuring airway patency and assessing vital signs, but also to obtain a careful history which may reveal such important evidence as alcoholism and liver disease, use of insulin, liability to convulsions, or past cardiac or renal disease. There should be a search for trauma about the patient's head or elsewhere on his body. Abnormal elevation or depression of blood pressure may be important as well as signs of systemic infection. Evidence of meningitis, such as neck stiffness, tends to diminish as coma deepens. Disturbances in respiration may be due to important pulmonary disease but may also represent a response to disturbed central nervous system function or systemic acid-base imbalance. Although evidence of focal cerebral or brainstem dysfunction may appear in the evolution of such systemic disturbances as hypoglycemia, the presence of persisting lateralizing or focal central nervous system signs in a comatose patient is in favor of a compressive or destructive lesion within the central nervous system. No matter what the cause, patients in coma may go through periods of decorticate and then decerebrate posturing, eventually reaching a stage of flaccid quadriplegia. However, in contrast to patients with destructive or severe depressive lesions of the brainstem, patients in metabolic coma tend to retain pupillary and oculovestibular reflexes.

Special investigations in the comatose patient are directed toward determining whether or not there is a local destructive lesion within the central nervous system, and if not, the nature of the responsible systemic disease.

Tests should include an echoencephalogram in case there should be a midline shift of supratentorial structures, skull x-ray, electrocardiogram, hemogram, blood glucose, serum electrolytes and bicarbonate, and arterial pH. Urine should be examined and samples of urine and blood kept for examination for toxic substances. Only if elevated intracranial pressure is considered to be absent should a lumbar puncture be performed. Examination of the cellular content of the cerebrospinal fluid will give important information in the presence of intracranial infection or hemorrhage. Evaluation of cerebrospinal fluid pH, osmolarity, and bicarbonate values may be of assistance in management of patients with protracted metabolic coma.

In the majority of these patients, autopsy findings are minimal in comparison to the gross clinical defects. The brain may be edematous, and there may be evidence of increased intracranial pressure. Neurons may exhibit changes suggestive of ischemic damage, and cell swelling may be prominent. It is clear, however, that neuronal dysfunction is far more important than are the morphologic changes.

In chronic hepatic failure, particularly in cirrhosis with extensive shunting of blood from the portal to systemic venous circulation, there is often prominent hypertrophy and hyperplasia of protoplasmic astrocytes (Fig. 4.10), particularly in the putamen, caudate nucleus, and cerebral cortex. Rarely, there may also be neuronal loss and cavitation in the putamen and caudate.

Hypoparathyroidism and familial pseudohypoparathyroidism both result in perivascular calcification in the brain, particularly in basal ganglia and dentate nuclei. The degree of calcification in the latter disease is often remarkable, and easily visualized by x-ray.

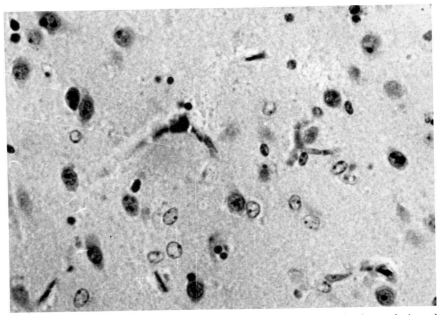

Figure 4.10. Hepatic encephalopathy. Astrocytes in the putamen exhibit hyperplasia and marked nuclear enlargement and vacuolation. (HE, × 300)

In uremic patients, the occurrence of a demyelinative peripheral neuropathy is well documented and appears distinct from any associated vitamin deficiency. The occurrence of a specific uremic encephalopathy is debatable; the findings of edema, hemorrhage, and infarction are most probably the result of associated hypertension.

REFERENCES

ADAMS, R. D., AND FOLEY, J. M. The neurological disorders associated with liver disease. *In* Metabolic and Toxic Diseases of the Nervous System. Association for Research in Nervous and Mental Diseases, Proceedings, Vol. 32. Ed. by H. H. Merritt and C. C. Hare. The Williams & Wilkins Co., Baltimore, 1953.

BRADY, R. O. Prenatal diagnosis of lipid storage diseases. Clin. Chem. 16:811, 1970.

CROME, L., AND STERN, J. The pathology of mental retardation. Little, Brown & Co., Boston, 1967.

FINCK, P. A. Exposure to carbon monoxide. Review of the literature and 567 autopsies. Milit. Med. 131:1513, 1966.

GRUNNETT, M. L. Changing incidence, distribution and histopathology of Wernicke's polioencephalopathy. Neurology (Minneap.) 19:1135, 1969.

HSIA, D. Y. The screening of hereditary metabolic defects among newborn infants. Canad. Med. Ass. J. 95:247, 1966.

LISS, L. Selective vulnerability of the central nervous system to anoxia. *In* Fifth International Congress of Neuropathology, Zurich, 1965. Ed. by Lüthy, F., and Bischoff, A. Excerpta Medica Foundation, New York, 1966.

MALAMUD, N. Neuropathology of phenylketonuria. J. Neuropath. Exp. Neurol. 25:254, 1966.

MENKES, J. H. The pathogenesis of mental retardation in phenylketonuria and other inborn errors of amino acid metabolism. Pediatrics 39:297, 1967.

MYERS, R. E., BEARD, R., AND ADAMSONS, K. Brain swelling in newborn rhesus monkey following prolonged partial asphyxia. Neurology (Minneap.) 19:1012, 1969.

O'BRIEN, J. S. Ganglioside-storage diseases. New Eng. J. Med. 284:893, 1971.

O'BRIEN, J. S., OKADA, S., CHEN, A., AND FILLERUP, D. L. Tay-Sachs disease. Detection of heterozygotes and homozygotes by serum hexosaminidase assay. New Eng. J. Med. 283: 15, 1970.

PLUM, F., AND POSNER, J. B. The Diagnosis of Stupor and Coma. F. A. Davis Co., Philadelphia, 1966.

ROBERTSON, D. M., WASAN, S. M., AND SKINNER, D. B. Ultrastructural features of early brainstem lesions of thiamine-deficient rats. Amer. J. Pathol. 52:1081, 1968.

ROSENBERG, L. E., AND SCRIVER, C. R. Disorders of amino acid metabolism. In Duncan's Diseases of Metabolism. 6th edition. Ed. by P. K. Bondy. W. B. Saunders Co., Philadelphia, 1969.

SHERLOCK, S. Hepatic coma. Gastroenterology 41:1, 1961.

SILVERMAN, D., MASLAND, R. L., SAUNDERS, M. G., AND SCHWAB, R. S. Irreversible coma associated with electrocerebral silence. Neurology (Minneap.) 20:525, 1970.

SLAGER, U. T., REILLY, E. B., AND BRANDT, R. A. The neuropathology of barbiturate intoxication. J. Neuropath. Exp. Neurol. 25:237, 1966.

SPILLANE, J. D. Nutritional Disorders of the Nervous System. E. & S. Livingstone, Ltd., Edinburgh, 1947.

VICTOR, M. The effects of nutritional deficiency on the nervous system. A comparison with the effects of carcinoma. In The Remote Effects of Cancer on the Nervous System. Ed. by The Late Lord Brain and F. H. Norris, Jr. Grune & Stratton, Inc., New York, 1965.

VOLK, B. W. (Ed). Tay-Sach's Disease. Grune & Stratton, Inc., New York and London, 1964.

WOOLF, L. I. Phenylketonuria: the relationship of phenotype to genotype. In Molecular Basis of Some Aspects of Mental Activity, Vol. 1. Ed. by O. Walaas. Academic Press, London, 1967.

ZIGLER, E. Familial mental retardation. A continuing dilemma. Science 155:292, 1967.

5

CEREBROVASCULAR DISEASE

INTRODUCTION

The brain constitutes only 2 percent of the body mass, but receives about 15 percent of the cardiac output and is responsible for 20 to 25 percent of the body's oxygen consumption at rest. The dependence of neural tissue on oxidative metabolism and the lack of significant stores of glycogen, coupled with the high metabolic rate, impose a requirement for essentially continuous perfusion and make the brain particularly vulnerable to interruption of blood flow. As previously discussed, the survival of ischemic or anoxic brain tissue varies in a regional fashion but is very limited as compared with most other tissues; hence the time available for the institution of therapeutic measures, even if effective, is very short indeed.

Vascular disease is by far the commonest cause of neurologic disability. At least 25 percent of all persons coming to autopsy have some evidence of cerebral damage secondary to vascular disease.

There are two principal ways in which vascular disease affects neural parenchyma; the blood flow may be inadequate, leading to ischemia with loss of function and necrosis, or a diseased vessel may burst to produce intracranial hemorrhage. In either case, there is relatively rapid evolution of a neurologic defect, commonly termed a "stroke." The nature of the resulting clinical disability reflects both the size and location of the parenchymal lesion, and ranges from mild transient disturbances to those which are rapidly fatal. It may present as any localized neural dysfunction.

The causes of strokes encompass the entire range of vascular disease. The cerebral vessels themselves may be at fault, as with malformations or atherosclerosis, or systemic factors, such as emboli from other sites or abnormalities of cardiac output, may be responsible. Although the list of responsible lesions is indeed a long one, it must be emphasized that in the brain, as elsewhere, atherosclerosis and the complications of hypertension are pre-eminent, and the cerebral involvement in these patients is usually accompanied by significant disease of the heart, kidneys, and other tissues.

ANATOMIC CONSIDERATIONS

The brain receives its blood supply through the carotid and vertebral arteries which anastomose through the circle of Willis at the base of the brain (Fig. 5.1). From the basal arteries arise the paramedian, short circumferential, and long circumferential arteries, the distribution of which are well described in standard textbooks of anatomy and neuroanatomy. A knowledge of the vascular pattern is, of course, essential in analyzing the patterns of cerebral infarction and the resulting clinical pictures.

Variation from the "anatomic" pattern is common and may determine the functional significance of occlusive disease in a large vessel. The posterior communicating and vertebral arteries are particularly prone to anatomic variations in size.

In addition to the circle of Willis, there are other anastomoses that may become important in the presence of occlusive vascular disease. Small vessels on the surface of the hemisphere in the boundary zones join the territories of supply of the three major cerebral arteries. Although they are seldom of a size to provide adequate collateral circulation in the event of occlusion of a major cerebral artery, they serve to

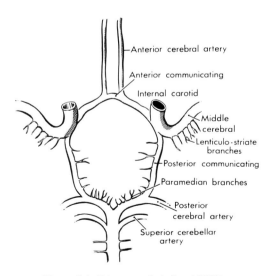

Figure 5.1. Diagram of circle of Willis.

limit the size of the infarct by nourishing the distal territory of supply. Thus, a cortical infarct following occlusion of the proximal middle cerebral artery is centered maximally in its proximal distribution about the Sylvian fissure but seldom extends to the edges of the territory of supply.

Anastomoses are also present between the deep penetrating arteries in the substance of the brain, but are of less importance. Significant arteriovenous shunts have not been demonstrated in the cerebral circulation.

Of more clinical significance are the anastomoses between branches of the external carotid arteries and intracranial vessels. Although usually inconspicuous in the normal individual, they are capable of dilatation following stenosis or occlusion of the internal carotid or vertebral arteries. Of particular importance are the anastomoses in the orbital fossa among branches of the ophthalmic, facial, and maxillary arteries, and in the posterior fossa with branches of the occipital arteries near the foramen magnum. The turbulent flow occurring in these dilated anastomoses may produce easily detected bruits, an important physical sign of disease in the major vessels. Paraxodically, patients who develop a prominent collateral circulation from the external circulation because of disease in the internal carotid arteries are more likely to have further strokes than those without such anastomotic development. This suggests that the cerebral circulation is in a particularly precarious situation if the circle of Willis is unable to shunt the necessary blood, producing the stimulus for other collateral channels to open.

PHYSIOLOGIC FACTORS

Physiologic factors combine with anatomic ones in determining the amount and distribution of cerebral blood flow. Total cerebral blood flow is determined primarily by the difference between the force of the systemic blood pressure and the resistance of the cerebral vessels. If cerebral vessels are not diseased, cerebral blood flow remains constant in spite of wide fluctuations in systemic pressure (autoregulation). Elevation of blood pressure leads to reactive vasoconstriction of cerebral vessels with an associated increase in cerebral vascular resistance. A fall in blood pressure produces cerebral vasodilatation. However, when the mean arterial pressure falls below 60 or 70 mm of mercury, the cerebral vessels are maximally dilated, autoregulation is lost, and flow then varies passively with systemic pressure. Elevation of venous or cerebrospinal fluid pressure also leads to cerebral vasodilatation.

Cerebral vessels respond also to chemical changes. Elevation of the $paCO_2$ produces dilatation of cerebral vessels. Because isolated pH changes in the blood do not alter cerebral vascular resistance, the vaso-dilatation which accompanies high $paCO_2$ presumably results from pH changes in tissue adjacent to brain arterioles. A fall in $paCO_2$ or the presence of oxygen in high concentrations leads to cerebral vasocon-striction and decreased cerebral blood flow.

Cerebral blood flow will alter to meet the metabolic requirements of the brain. In normal circumstances cerebral blood flow is regulated to maintain an average arteriovenous oxygen difference of seven volumes percent at a $paCO_2$ of 40 mm of mercury, but if the metabolic needs of the brain increase, there will be a proportionate increase in cerebral blood flow. Conversely, if cerebral metabolism is reduced, as with gen-eral anesthesia or myxedema, there will be a reduction in total cerebral blood flow. Following destruction of brain tissue, as occurs with an ischemic infarct, there may be local tissue acidosis leading to dilatation of cerebral vessels near the damaged region. This may divert blood from marginally damaged areas to regions of irreversible tissue necrosis (cere-bral "centripetal" steal syndrome).

In diseases such as polycythemia, the viscosity of the blood is ele-vated, raising the resistance to flow and thereby reducing cerebral blood flow. Polycythemic patients also have a tendency to thrombo-embolism and frequently develop ischemic cerebral vascular damage.

ISCHEMIC CEREBROVASCULAR DISEASE

Ischemic cerebrovascular disease affects the individual in one or more of the following ways: (1) transient ischemic attacks; (2) completed stroke; (3) stroke-in-evolution.

Transient Ischemic Attacks

Transient ischemic attacks are episodes of reversible neurologic def-icit lasting from a few minutes to a few hours, resulting from inadequate local cerebral blood flow. Current usage limits the duration of symp-toms arbitrarily to 24 hours or less.

A patient may have one or many attacks, with the nature of the symp-toms depending upon which arterial supply has been comprised. Trans-ient aphasia, hemiparesis, and hemianesthesia including the face or hemianopic visual field defect, point to ischemia of the cerebral hemi-spheres. Dysarthria, diplopia, or sudden weakness of both legs is found with brainstem ischemia. Vertigo is less specific and may appear with dysfunction of either brainstem or cerebral hemispheres. It is common for a patient to experience repeated attacks which are almost identical in nature. A change in the symptoms of the attack is suggestive of changing or evolving injury. A patient with ischemic attacks related to one internal carotid artery may eventually develop additional symptoms pointing to ischemia arising from the opposite carotid or the basilar artery. Occasionally, the original attacks will cease entirely. It also seems likely that patients may experience undetected ischemic attacks in clinically "silent" areas of the brain.

Eventually, 60 percent of patients with recurrent cerebral ischemia arising from the internal carotid artery and 40 percent of those with vertebrobasilar ischemia will proceed to a completed stroke in the region involved in the ischemic attack. Patients with episodes of cerebral ischemia who develop a completed stroke usually do so within 1 to 3 years of the onset of ischemic symptoms. Therefore, the patient with symptoms of cerebral ischemia merits careful assessment, often including such investigative procedures as angiography.

Although aphasia or diplopia may be of localizing value in terms of the region of brain structure involved in an ischemic attack, it is usually difficult on clinical grounds alone to conclude where the significant site or sites of vascular damage are located. For instance, an occluded internal carotid artery may become symptomatic only after collateral circulation through the circle of Willis is impaired by additional thrombosis in a vertebral artery. Aphasia, indicating ischemia in the posterior frontal region of the leading hemisphere for speech, might be due to narrowing in the middle cerebral artery, emboli reaching that artery, an occlusion in the ipsilateral carotid artery, contralateral carotid disease, or a combination of these lesions.

The important factors of hypertension, anti-hypertensive drug therapy, obesity, diabetes mellitus, smoking, cardiac disease, especially congestive failure, and hematopoietic diseases should be assessed because they serve to influence the severity of vascular disease and may be remediable.

Neck bruits in the adult imply turbulent flow due usually to stenosis of the vessel lumen. The disappearance of a bruit suggests that a previously narrowed artery has become completely occluded.

Retinal arterial pressure, as measured by the technique of opthalmodynamometry, may be lower in the eye on the side of a carotid occlusion. A thermal probe may show lowered forehead temperature on the side of extracranial vascular disease. The measurement of total and regional cerebral blood flow using radioactive tracers has provided important new information about cerebrovascular disease but remains primarily a research method at this time.

Angiography is a radiologic method whereby the location and nature of extracranial and intracranial vascular lesions can be demonstrated, and is used when there is diagnostic doubt or an indication for vascular surgery.

Although some patients complain of symptoms immediately after standing up or twisting their neck, it is often very difficult to reproduce this phenomenon purposefully. Manual compression of the carotid artery in an attempt to reproduce symptoms is hazardous and has led to completed strokes.

Completed Stroke

Completed stroke refers to a stable neurologic deficit due to vascular disease which may be thrombotic, embolic, or hemorrhagic.

Ischemic strokes can appear in patients with no previous history of cerebrovascular disease but often they follow upon one or more transient ischemic attacks. It is usually impossible to differentiate clinically between an embolic or thrombotic stroke unless there are associated findings which favor embolism, such as cardiac valvular disease, a change in cardiac rhythm, or the presence of emboli in other organs. Both embolic and thrombotic strokes may begin suddenly, and, although there may be premonitory symptoms, the neurologic deficit is often complete within a few minutes. Systolic blood pressure drops during sleep and this may be a factor contributing to the high incidence of completed strokes developing at that time.

As with transient ischemic attacks, obvious precipitating factors are often absent although occasionally a history of marked rotation or extension of the neck or hypotension secondary to silent myocardial infarction can be identified. Headache is often present at the outset and may result from the dilatation of collateral vessels. Loss of consciousness indicates a massive hemisphere lesion, damage to the brainstem, or markedly increased intracranial pressure due to cerebral edema. Mild confusion or unsteadiness may be followed by heaviness and tingling down one side of the body. Symptoms usually progress quickly, and, within a few minutes of the appearance of dizziness, the patient may have nearly complete paralysis with or without additional localizing manifestations. By the time a physician sees the patient, neurologic damage is generally complete and attention is directed toward prevention of complications and rehabilitation.

Stroke-in-Evolution

A minority of patients develop a stroke which evolves slowly over many hours. An initial weakness or sensory disturbance may change little in the first few hours but eventually the neurologic deficit increases.

This gradual evolution may be due to a slow extension of a thrombus, the gradual development of cerebral edema, or thrombus formation beginning at the site of embolic impaction. In theory at least, these factors can be modified by appropriate therapy.

PATHOLOGY OF ISCHEMIC CEREBROVASCULAR DISEASE

The interpretation of the clinical and pathologic features in cases of ischemic cerebrovascular disease is based on the interaction of two more or less independent variables:

(1) The nature and location of the changes in the vessels, having regard to the vascular pattern in that individual.

(2) The nature and size of the changes in cerebral tissue, and the specific areas, nuclei, and tracts affected.

For example, occlusion of the internal carotid artey at the bifurcation is often symptomless. However, others will suffer minor or massive cerebral infarction with permanent residual deficits, or display evidence of recurrent transient ischemia. Local vascular factors, such as the anatomic configuration, acquired collateral circulation, disease in collateral vessels, and such systemic factors as cardiac output, blood pressure, oxygen content, and viscosity of blood will interact to determine the effects on the brain of any given vascular lesion.

Vascular Lesions

The cerebral vessels are subject to the same vascular malformations, inflammations, and degenerations as those in the remainder of the body. Current opinion holds that 60 percent of ischemic cerebrovascular disease is due to atherosclerosis and its complications, 30 percent is due to emboli (usually thromboemboli arising from the heart), with the 5 to 10 percent remaining the result of other vascular diseases.

Occasionally, no organic occlusive vascular disease is found to account for cerebral infarction. In some of these instances, emboli or thrombi which have undergone lysis may have been the cause. In other cases, a drop in blood pressure may have reduced flow beyond a stenotic area below the critical level. Following subarachnoid hemorrhage, severe arterial spasm may be demonstrated angiographically and is considered by many to be a cause of infarction. There is also some evidence that spasm of small vessels may produce the cortical microinfarcts frequently found in severe (malignant) hypertension. The development of sudden severe hypertension may lead to the symptoms of hypertensive encephalopathy, characterized by headache, drowsiness, seizures, and focal neurologic signs. The sudden increase in intraluminal vascular pressure leads to a combination of cerebral edema and areas of focal reflex vasoconstriction and ischemia.

Atherosclerosis has a definite predilection for certain locations. The carotid bifurcation, proximal and distal portions of the internal carotid arteries, the proximal portion of the middle cerebral arteries, the upper end of the vertebral arteries, and the basilar artery are most frequently the sites of stenotic plaques and the complicating lesions of thrombosis and intimal hemorrhage (Figs. 5.2, 5.3). In contrast, the an-

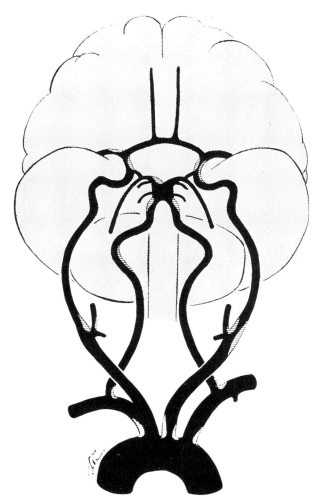

Figure 5.2. Schematic diagram of the cerebral blood supply, showing the common locations of clinically significant atherosclerosis (*shaded areas*).

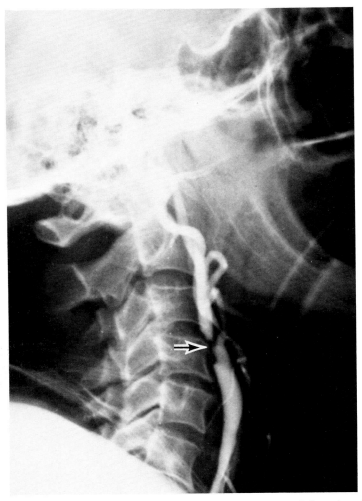

Figure 5.3. Angiogram showing extreme atherosclerotic narrowing of the point of origin of the internal carotid artery (*arrow*). Patient complained of intermittent episodes of numbness and weakness of hand and arm on the opposite side of the body.

terior cerebral artery is seldom severely involved, and an infarct in its territory is more often due to embolism. As in other arteries such as the aorta, local hemodynamic factors have been implicated in explaining this regional disparity, but the factors responsible for localization of plaques remain basically unknown.

In the presence of hypertension, small perforating arteries and arterioles share the reactions of vessels of similar size in the kidneys and elsewhere and may show medial degeneration, hyalinization, hyperplastic sclerosis, and fibrinoid necrosis. These small vessel changes may be responsible for ischemic lesions or hemorrhages (*vide infra*). Small perforating vessels rarely show occlusion when there are infarcts within their territory of supply; more often plaques or thrombosis in the parent vessel produce narrowing or occlusion of their ostia.

Cerebral Ischemic Lesions

Cerebral Infarction

The size and location of cerebral infarcts are dependent on the vascular factors outlined above. Infarcts may be in any part of the brain but the majority are in the territory of supply of the middle cerebral artery (Fig. 5.4) and the vertebral-basilar system. Small infarcts are found in about 25 percent of elderly individuals at autopsy, but many of these were associated with little or no clinical deficit.

A large infarct becomes apparent grossly in about 24 hours as a region of swelling, hyperemia, and slight softening. Small hemorrhages are often present and are occasionally quite severe when an occluding embolus has shifted or undergone lysis, or spasm has passed off and permitted return of blood flow to the necrotic area (hemorrhagic infarction). During the ensuing several days this tissue becomes progressively more swollen, soft, and friable (Figs. 5.5, 5.6, 5.7). The swelling of the necrotic tissue and adjacent viable tissue plays a major role in elevation of intracranial pressure and in the progression of signs following large infarcts, and may produce tentorial herniation with secondary brainstem compression.

In the ensuing weeks, the necrotic tissue becomes liquefied (Fig. 5.8) and gradually disappears, leaving behind a fluid-filled cavity containing a few cobweb-like strands of vessels with adherent glial and connective tissue (Fig. 5.9). Wallerian and trans-synaptic degeneration are found in the appropriate tracts and nuclei.

The earliest microscopic change, visible in 6 to 12 hours, is coagulation necrosis ("ischemic cell change"), best seen at first in the larger neurons, but involving all tissue elements except for occasional sparing of endothelial and microglial cells (Fig. 5.10). Myelin sheaths rapidly become swollen, irregular, and globular, and axons swell and fragment.

Neutrophilic leukocytes appear near vessels and in the overlying meninges during the first and second days, but are usually few in number and rapidly undergo lysis. Macrophages are responsible for most of the phagocytosis and digestion of the necrotic tissue. They are derived at first from the microglial and perivascular cells in the vicinity of

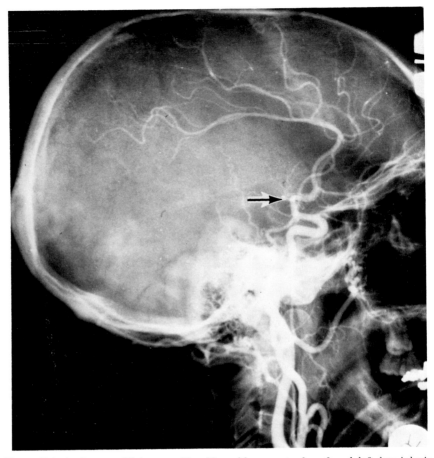

Figure 5.4. Angiogram. Male, age 47, with sudden onset of profound left hemiplegia, leading to death 6 days later. There is good filling of carotid and anterior cerebral arteries. No dye has entered the middle cerebral artery or its branches, as a result of complete occlusion at its origin (*arrow*). The occlusion was the result of an embolus from a left ventricular mural thrombus overlying a myocardial infarct.

the infarct and later from circulating monocytes. As they accumulate cellular and myelin debris, their cytoplasm becomes distended with digestive vacuoles containing lipids in various stages of breakdown and pigments from phagocytosis of erythrocytes (gitter cell or compound granular corpuscle). Removal of the necrotic debris from a large infarct is a rather slow process and remnants of dead tissue, surrounded by macrophages, may persist for many months.

Astrocytes at the edges of the infarct undergo conspicuous hyper-

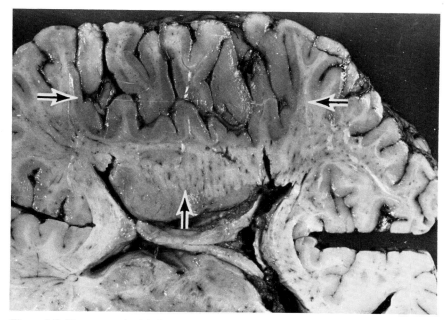

Figure 5.5. Recent cerebral infarct. The necrotic tissue appears swollen and discolored. The area of infarction (*arrows*) corresponds to a large portion of the territory of the middle cerebral artery, including its deep branches; the occlusion was near its origin.

trophy and hyperplasia beginning on about the third day, and during the ensuing weeks a moderately dense glial scar develops around the cavity (Fig. 5.11). There is some meningeal fibrosis over the infarct but little collagen is formed elsewhere except along vessels within and adjacent to the cavity.

Microinfarction

Severe sclerosis, fibrinoid necrosis, inflammation, embolism, intravascular coagulation, and (perhaps) spasm involving arterioles and small perforating arteries produce multiple small infarcts widely distributed throughout the brain. In the cortex these often appear as narrow linear strips perpendicular to the surface, corresponding to the territories of supply of vessels entering the cortex from the meninges. Because they are so small, resorption of the necrotic tissue is followed by a contracted glial scar without much cavitation (Fig. 5.12). When these small infarcts are numerous, the external surface of the cortex may assume a granular appearance, analogous to the granularity imparted to the renal cortex by small vessel disease. In white matter and particularly

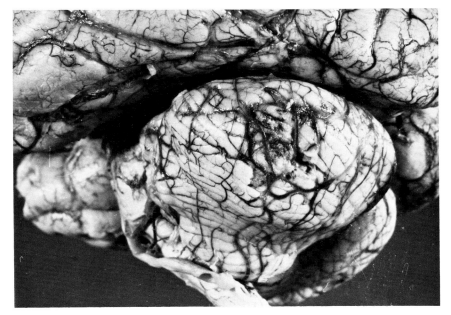

Figure 5.6. Small recent cerebellar infarct in the distal territory of the posterior inferior cerebellar artery, showing focal hemorrhage and softening. Embolus from mitral vegetation.

in putamen and globus pallidus, the loss of tissue is usually in a perivascular distribution leaving perivascular "lacunes" (Fig. 5.13) surrounded by glial scar and containing occasional macrophages.

The microinfarcts are, taken singly, of very little clinical significance, but when numerous or accumulative over a period of time they may well produce progressive cortical dysfunction or progressive rigidity and dyskinesia and a flexed posture. Small vessel disease in the cortex in older age groups may lead to sufficient neuronal loss to produce a demented state.

Transient Ischemic Attacks

The pathogenesis of short-lived episodes of focal cerebral ischemia is far from clear, but several factors are known to play a role. In a few cases, small emboli ("microemboli") of platelets or of atheromatous debris may be seen passing slowly through the retinal arterioles during attacks of monocular blindness (Fig. 5.14). These emboli often arise from ulcerated atheromas in the large vessels of the neck. Transient ischemic attacks may also be assiciated with severe stenosing atherosclerosis of the large vessels, and may occur under circumstances, such as rapid postural change, when blood pressure may be transiently reduced. In other instances, thrombosis of a vessel may have produced focal non-infarctive ischemia followed by collateral dilatation and restoration of blood flow. Reversal of flow in an anastomotic circulation is another, rather uncommon cause. For example, in the subclavian steal syndrome, stenosis of the subclavian artery proximal to the origin of the vertebral artery may cause a fall in pressure beyond the stenosis leading to reversal of flow down the vertebral artery with resultant brainstem ischemia, especially when the arm on the involved side is exercised.

Infarcts of the Spinal Cord

These are very much less common than those of the brain because of the segmental blood supply and very rich anastomatic circulation of the spinal cord, and the infrequency of significant atherosclerosis of the spinal arteries. A dissecting aortic aneurysm may obliterate the origins of intercostal and lumbar arteries. Small emboli occasionally enter the

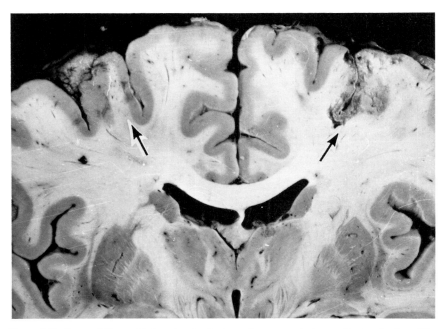

Figure 5.7. Recent bilateral infarction in the boundary zones between the territories of the anterior and middle cerebral arteries (*arrows*), the result of a brief period of cardiac arrest in a patient with severe atherosclerotic narrowing of cerebral vessels.

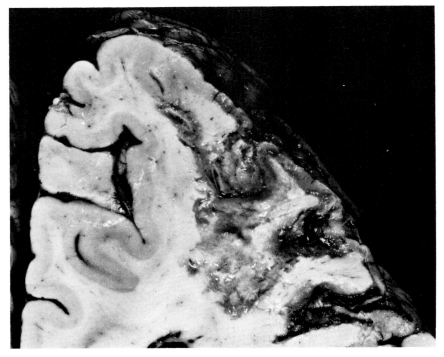

Figure 5.8. Lateral parieto-occipital infarct, 3 weeks duration, showing liquefaction of necrotic tissue.

spinal circulation, and spinal arteries are sometimes involved in generalized vasculitis. Compression of the anterior spinal or radicular arteries may produce some of the spinal cord destruction found with cervical intervertebral disc disease.

Venous Infarction

As in other tissues and organs, infarcts following venous occlusion are usually characterized by severe hemorrhage and edema of the necrotic tissue. Although uncommon, there are three important causes: trauma (including surgical trauma), local infection of bone or meninges leading to thrombophlebitis, and dehydration (especially in infants). Thrombosis in the major dural sinuses or their larger venous tributaries usually results in hemorrhagic infarction.

SPONTANEOUS INTRACRANIAL HEMORRHAGE

The term "spontaneous" is used to identify those intracranial hemorrhages which are not due to head injury. Spontaneous intracranial

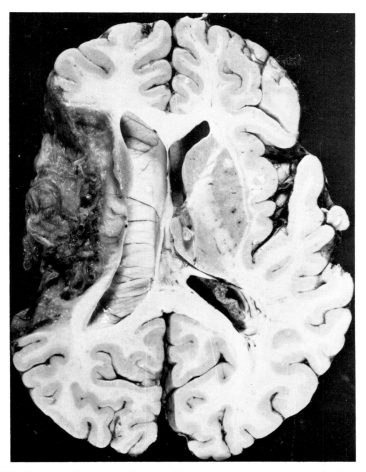

Figure 5.9. Cerebral infarct, several years old. A large cavity occupies much of the middle cerebral artery distribution.

hemorrhage may occur within the substance of the brain (intracerebral hemorrhage) or into the meninges, most commonly subarachnoid bleeding. The hemorrhage may range in size from a few inconsequential petechiae to massively destructive and rapidly lethal hematomas. This section will be concerned with the commoner forms of major hemorrhage which constitute about 10 percent of all "strokes."

The majority of such hemorrhages are those occurring in association with hypertension and those following rupture of arterial berry aneurysms. Less common are those occurring in relation to platelet and coagulation defects, often as a terminal event in patients with leukemias,

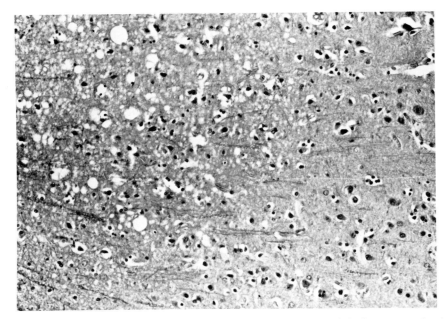

Figure 5.10. Edge of recent cerebral infarct. Tissue at the *upper left* shows necrosis of cells and edema. There is as yet no significant cellular reaction. (Luxol fast blue-hematoxylin-eosin (LFB-HE), × 130)

lymphomas, or bone marrow depression. Other important causes of hemorrhage include rupture of mycotic, arteriosclerotic, or dissecting aneurysms of intracranial vessels, arteritis, vascular malformations involving brain or meninges, and hemorrhage into primary or metastatic tumors.

Hypertensive Intracerebral Hemorrhage

Massive intracerebral hemorrhage is a major and often lethal complication of hypertension. In Canada from 1950 to 1964, the mortality from hypertensive cerebral hemorrhage declined by 21 percent, suggesting that effective therapy of hypertension reduces the incidence of hemorrhage.

Small cerebral arteries and arterioles in hypertensive patients show medial atrophy and hyalinization, hyperplasia, and occasionally necrosis similar to that seen in vessels elsewhere in the body. The source of bleeding is generally thought to be the rupture of a weakened segment in such a vessel. Small thin-walled saccular or fusiform outpouchings (Charcot-Bouchard aneurysms) occur along small perforating arteries, apparently arising in areas of focal medial degeneration, and are prob-

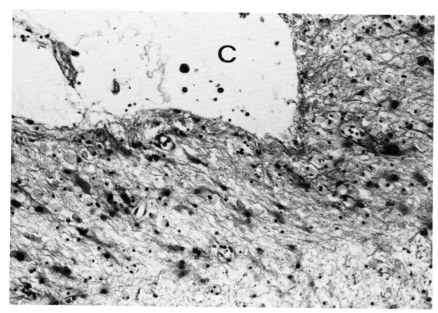

Figure 5.11. Old cerebral infarct. The wall of the cavity (*C*) is formed of glial scar tissue. (LFB-HE, × 350)

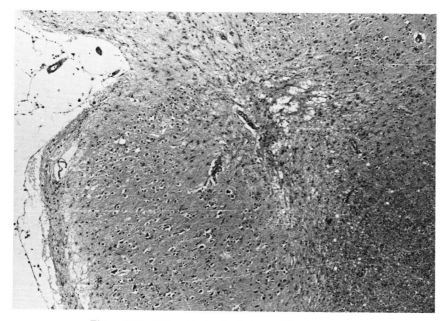

Figure 5.12. Old cortical microinfarct. (LFB-HE, × 50)

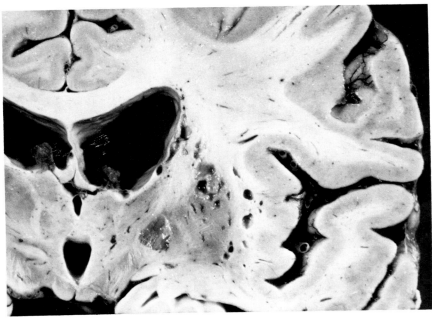

Figure 5.13. Multiple small old infarcts in basal ganglia and internal capsule. Note dilatation of ipsilateral ventricle.

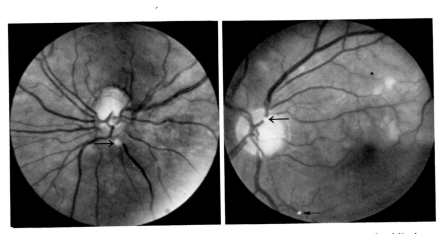

Figure 5.14. Fundus photographs from two patients with transient monocular blindness (amaurosis fugax). *A (left):* dull white platelet embolus (*arrow*). *B (right):* two shiny refractile atheromatous emboli (*arrows*).

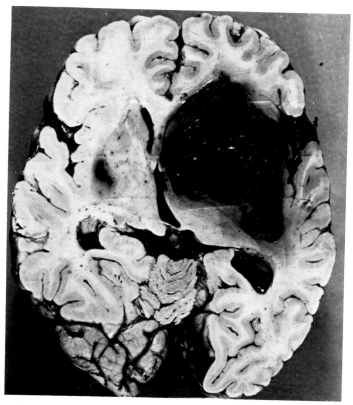

Figure 5.15. Large hypertensive intracerebral hemorrhage involving basal ganglia and internal capsule. There is a small putaminal hemorrhage on the opposite side as well.

ably the source of most hemorrhages. Occasionally there is convincing evidence that massive bleeding has occurred into an area of recent infarction, presumably because of the local vascular damage.

Intracerebral hemorrhage frequently occurs during a period of physical activity or stress when blood pressure may be higher than usual. Symptoms usually begin abruptly and may be those of increased intracranial pressure, meningeal irritation, and focal destruction of brain. Clinical signs may progress for a period of hours as bleeding continues to dissect and destroy brain tissue and elevation of intracranial pressure leads to loss of consciousness.

About 80 percent of hypertensive hemorrhages are in the cerebral hemispheres, and of these, about 75 percent originate in the lateral basal ganglia, notably the putamen, where degenerative vascular changes and microaneurysms of perforating arteries are generally most evident (Fig. 5.15). Next in frequency are those in the thalamus and in the white matter of the hemispheres (Fig. 5.16). The pons and cerebellar hemispheres each account for about 10 percent. In the pons, bleeding often begins near the junction of the basis pontis and the tegmentum. Cerebellar hemorrhage arises most frequently in or near the dentate nucleus.

Intracerebral hemorrhages are usually large, although in the brainstem a volume of 10 ml may be lethal. They produce laceration and massive distortion in the adjacent tissues and usually result in large intracranial displacements. Secondary hemorrhages around the hematoma and in the upper brainstem are common. The hemorrhage frequently ruptures into an adjacent ventricle or less often directly into the subarachnoid space, but until this occurs the cerebrospinal fluid may be deceptively free of red cells and thus of little help in distinguishing hemorrhage from infarction.

Small hemorrhages, usually slit-like in configuration, are occasionally found in superficial subcortical white matter or basal ganglia, either as

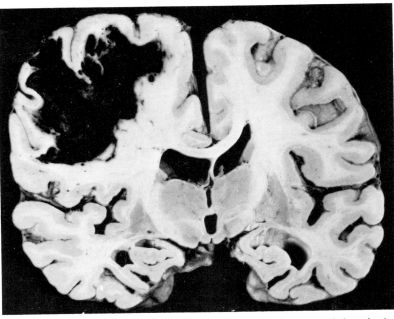

Figure 5.16. Hemorrhage into centrum semiovale in an elderly man with lymphatic leukemia and depression of platelets. Note also the severe temporal lobe atrophy, the result of Alzheimer's disease.

recent occurrences, or after resorption as irregular hemosiderin-stained cavities.

Most major hemorrhages produce death before there is much tissue response. The early reaction is that of edema of adjacent tissues and exudation of a few neutrophils. Later, macrophages undertake the slow process of phagocytosis and digestion and the resultant cavity is walled off by a scar which usually contains a fairly prominent collagenous component in addition to astrocytes. Hemosiderin-laden macrophages may persist in the brain for many years. As with any destructive lesion, the involved tracts and nuclei will exhibit the appropriate secondary changes.

Berry Aneurysms

Berry aneurysms are saccular outpouchings, usually 5 to 10 mm in diameter occurring most often at points of bifurcation along the large arteries comprising the circle of Willis and its proximal branches (Fig. 5.17). Unfortunately, they are relatively common, being found in about 2 percent of autopsies and, most often (75 percent), after they have ruptured to produce fatal hemorrhage. Their etiology is uncertain. It is widely held that they occur on the basis of a developmental defect in the media in which there remains a small gap bridged only by intima and

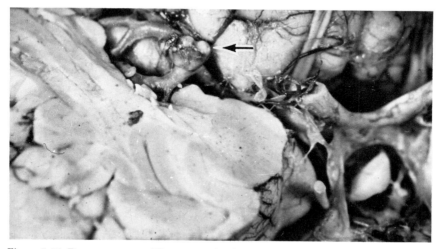

Figure 5.17. Berry aneurysm. The temporal pole has been removed to show the course of the middle cerebral artery in the Sylvian fissure. The aneurysm (*arrow*) is located at the first major branching of the artery, and shows two thin-walled blisters at its fundus. The upper end of the internal carotid artery and the origins of the anterior cerebral and posterior communicating arteries are at the *right*.

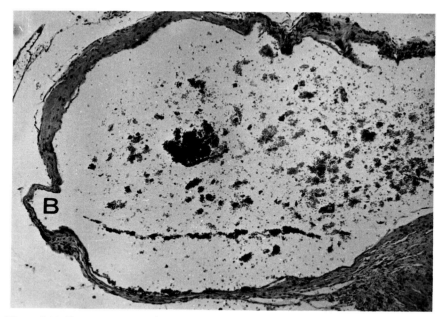

Figure 5.18. Berry aneurysm. A portion of the wall of the vessel of origin is at the *lower right*. The wall is composed almost solely of a thin layer of fibrous tissue; note the marked thinness of the "blister" (*B*) at the fundus. (Hematoxylin-eosin (HE), × 45)

adventitia on the inner aspect of the fork of bifurcation. Such gaps are frequently found in otherwise normal cerebral vessels. Over a period of years, pressure within the artery and degeneration of elastica at the bifurcation result in herniation of the intima through the gap to produce a thin-walled sac (Fig. 5.18) which enlarges and eventually ruptures. The role of degenerative and atrophic changes in media and elastica at the site is heavily emphasized by some; others have suggested that a localized destructive inflammation may be involved. Still others have proposed that the initial small blisters represent vestiges of branches that underwent incomplete involution during embryogenesis, leaving medial gaps at their points of origin.

Thus, although the defect giving rise to the aneurysm is probably intra-uterine in origin (hence the term, "congenital saccular aneurysm"), it must be emphasized that the aneurysms are seldom, if ever, present at birth; they are occasionally found during the first decade, but are usually of significance in middle-aged and elderly individuals. Hypertension is present in about half the patients. Elevated intraluminal pressure apparently promotes enlargement and rupture of the aneurysm. There is an unexplained high incidence in persons with poly-cystic renal disease, perhaps related again to associated hypertension.

Sites of Aneurysms

Any point of branching along the major cerebral arteries at the base of the brain may be the site of an aneurysm, but 85 percent occur on the circle of Willis, the common sites being: (1) anterior cerebral-anterior communicating junction; (2) first major branching of the middle cerebral artery in the Sylvian fissure; (3) at the origin of the posterior communicating artery from the internal carotid artery; (4) at the bifurcation of the internal carotid artery into anterior and middle cerebral arteries.

The posterior fossa vessels account for about 15 percent, the common sites being the upper end of the basilar artery and the origin of the posterior inferior cerebellar artery from the vertebral artery.

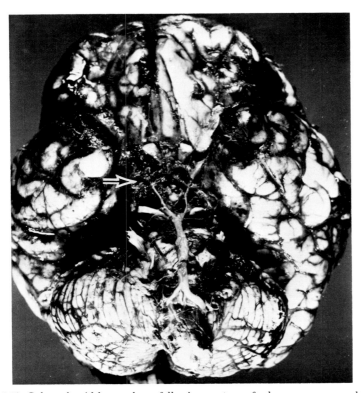

Figure 5.19. Subarachnoid hemorrhage following rupture of a berry aneurysm which was located at the internal carotid-posterior communicating artery junction (*arrow*). The aneurysm sac was largely destroyed by the hemorrhage.

In about 20 percent of cases, more than one aneurysm is present, often symmetrically located.

Manifestations of Berry Aneurysms

Local Pressure. Rarely, the aneurysm may become several centimeters in diameter, compressing and distorting adjacent tissues, particularly the optic pathways and hypothalamus, leading to symptoms of a slowly expanding space-occupying mass. Small aneurysms may be strategically located in such a way as to produce focal signs. Notable in this regard is isolated third nerve paralysis occasionally produced by compression by a carotid-posterior communicating aneurysm. In most cases, however, the first clinical evidence of the aneurysm's presence is following rupture.

Hemorrhage. Rupture of an aneurysm floods the subarachnoid space with blood (Fig. 5.19), producing the clinical picture of sudden, very severe headache, often likened to a blow to the head and frequently followed by transient unconsciousness. In 60 to 70 percent of patients, the blood tears through the adjacent pia into the brain, producing an intracerebral hematoma with laceration and compression of the adjacent tissue, and may result in localizing signs as well as meningeal irritation. Less often, the blood tears through the outer layer of arachnoid to produce a subdural hematoma. Usually, the clinician requires the assistance of cerebral angiography to be certain of the location of the ruptured aneurysm (Fig. 5.20).

An aneurysm may at first leak only small amounts of blood, producing mild headache, the "warning leaks," seen in perhaps 50 percent of patients. A massive hemorrhage leads to rapid elevation of intracranial pressure reflected as papilledema, retinal hemorrhages, nausea, drowsiness, confusion, and coma.

The first hemorrhage is massively destructive and fatal in about 30 percent of instances. Of the remainder, about half will have repeated hemorrhage within a few days or weeks. Surgery to clip or otherwise obliterate the aneurysm is primarily directed at preventing additional hemorrhages in those individuals who have survived the initial event.

Infarction. The initial cerebral damage is often complicated by the occurrence of ischemic necrosis adjacent to the site of hemorrhage, and occasionally of large areas of cerebral cortex. The mechanism is debated, but recent angiographic studies have emphasized the occurrence of spasm in large vessels near, and occasionally remote from, the aneurysm. Other factors leading to ischemic damage include stretching and distortions of vessels by accumulated blood in the subarachnoid space, pre-existent atherosclerosis, hypotension, and peri-

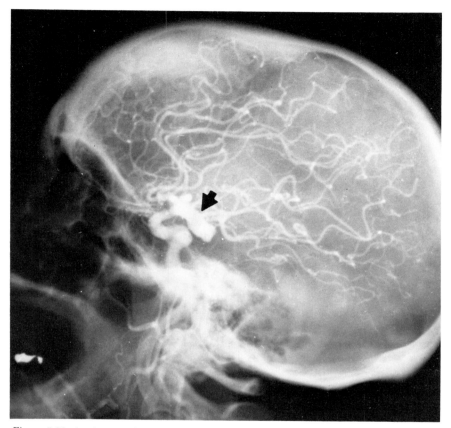

Figure 5.20. Angiogram showing a large berry aneurysm (*arrow*) arising from the internal carotid artery at the origin of the posterior communicating artery. The patient was an 82 year old man who presented with a unilateral third nerve palsy of 3 days' duration, followed by sudden coma.

vascular sheath hemorrhages, and, occasionally, vascular occlusions produced at the time of surgery.

Meningeal Fibrosis. The breakdown of blood in the subarchnoid space incites fibrosis of the meninges which occasionally is of sufficient severity to obstruct the flow of cerebrospinal fluid and produce hydrocephalus as a late complication.

REFERENCES

CARTER, A. B. Cerebral Infarction. Oxford University Press, London, 1964.

CASTAIGNE, P., LHERMITTE, F., GAUTIER, J.-C., ESCOUROLLE, R., AND DEROUESNÉ, C. Internal carotid artery occlusion. A study of 61 instances in 50 patients with postmortem data. Brain 93:231, 1970.

COLE, F. M., AND YATES, P. O. The occurrence and significance of intracerebral microaneurysms. J. Path. Bact. 93:393, 1967.

CROMPTON, M. R. The pathogenesis of cerebral infarction following the rupture of cerebral berry aneurysms. Brain 87:491, 1964.

CROMPTON, M. R. The pathogenesis of cerebral aneurysms. Brain 89:797, 1966.

DINSDALE, H. B. Spontaneous hemorrhage in the posterior fossa. Arch. Neurol. (Chicago) 10:200, 1964.

FIELDS, W. S., AND SAHS, A. L. (Eds). Intracranial Aneurysms and Subarachnoid Hemorrhage. Charles C Thomas, Publisher, Inc., Springfield, Ill., 1965.

FRIEDMAN, G. D., WILSON, W. S., MOSIER, J. M., COLANDREA, M. A., AND NICHAMAN, M. Z. Transient ischemic attacks in a community. J. A. M. A. 210:1428, 1969.

GORDON, P. C. The epidemiology of cerebral vascular disease in Canada: an analysis of mortality data. Canad. Med. Ass. J. 95:1004, 1966.

HARPER, A. M. Autoregulation of cerebral blood flow: influence of the arterial blood pressure on the blood flow through the cerebral cortex. J. Neurol. Neurosurg. Psychiat. 29:398, 1966.

KANE, W. C., AND ARONSON, S. M. Cardiac disorders predisposing to embolic stroke. Stroke 1:164, 1970.

KANNEL, W. B., DAWBER, T. R., COHEN, M. E., AND McNAMARA, P. M. Vascular disease of the brain. Epidemiologic aspects: the Framingham study. Amer. J. Public Health 55:1355, 1965.

MARSHALL, J. The Management of Cerebrovascular Disease. 2nd edition. J. & A. Churchill, Ltd., London, 1968.

McBRIEN, D. J., BRADLEY, R. D., AND ASHTON, N. The nature of retinal emboli in stenosis of the internal carotid artery. Lancet 1:697, 1963.

MILLIKAN, C. H., SIEKERT, R. G., AND WHISNANT, J. P. (Eds). Cerebral Vascular Diseases. Grune & Stratton, Inc., New York and London, 1966.

MOOSSY, J. Cerebral infarction and intracranial arterial thrombosis. Arch. Neurol. (Chicago) 14:119, 1966.

MUTLU, N., BERRY, R. G., AND ALPERS, B. J. Massive cerebral hemorrhage. Clinical and pathological correlations. Arch. Neurol. (Chicago) 8:644, 1963.

REIVICH, M. Regulation of the cerebral circulation. In Proceedings of the Congress of Neurological Surgeons, Vol. 16. Ed. by R. G. Ojemann. The Williams & Wilkins Co., Baltimore, 1969.

RUSSELL, R. W. R. Observations on intracerebral aneurysms. Brain 86:425, 1963.

THEANDER, S., AND GRANHOLM, L. Sequelae after spontaneous subarachnoid hemorrhage, with special reference to hydrocephalus and Korsakoff's syndrome. Acta Neurol. Scand. 43:479, 1967.

WALTON, J. N. Subarachnoid Hemorrhage. E. & S. Livingstone, Ltd. Edinburgh, 1956.

6

DEMYELINATING DISEASES

INTRODUCTION

The descriptive term "demyelinating disease" was introduced in 1868 by Charcot, and has been the subject of changing definitions as more has been learned about some of the diseases placed in this category.

Myelin sheaths are the highly specialized processes of interfascicular oligodendroglia in the central nervous system. and of Schwann cells in the peripheral nervous system. They are vulnerable to injury of many types for example, with ischemia, or trauma, and will also disintegrate if the contained axon is lost for any reason. In addition, however, there is a group of conditions in which it appears that the primary point of damage is the myelin-forming cell and/or the myelin sheath, with the axonal changes, phagocytosis, and gliosis being secondary phenomena. These are the demyelinating diseases.

This chapter is concerned with those diseases in which there has been apparently normal myelination of the nervous system, but later, myelin is damaged and disintegrates with relative sparing of other tissue elements. Multiple sclerosis and acute disseminated encephalomyelitis are two important diseases in this group. Recent evidence indicates that parainfectious neuritis and the Landry-Guillain-Barré syndrome are also primarily demyelinative in nature. Experimental allergic encephalomyelitis and experimental allergic neuropathy, models of demyelinative diseases which show similarities to human disease, are described briefly at the end of this chapter.

A number of diffuse white matter diseases, collectively known as the leukodystrophies, are due to inborn errors of metabolism (known or postulated), which interfere with normal myelination or myelin turnover ("dysmyelinating diseases"). They are discussed in Chapter 4.

MULTIPLE SCLEROSIS

Multiple sclerosis is a chronic and usually relapsing disease of the central nervous system which commonly begins in early adult life and is characterized by symptoms and signs pointing to multiple episodes of randomly located lesions of the central nervous system. In spite of its pleomorphic nature and the lack of diagnostic laboratory tests, clinical diagnosis is usually not long in doubt.

Epidemiology and Etiology

In spite of intensive study, the etiology remains unknown. However, a number of features of the disease are compatible with its being an infective process.

The risk of developing symptoms increases with age until 30 years and then decreases steadily, possibly reflecting chance exposure in early life to a noxious agent with a long latent period before lesions occur. The incidence of the disease varies greatly in different geographic regions of the world, and is related to latitude. In North America and Europe, the frequency of the disease increases as one moves northward, with maximum incidence between latitudes 45 and 50 degrees, but no consistent evidence of increasing frequency north of 50 degrees. The incidence of the disease in Winnipeg is 3 times greater than in New Orleans and the mortality rate is 5 times as great. The latitude factor also operates in the southern hemisphere so that the hospitalization rate for the disease is greater in the South Island than in the North Island of New Zealand. A low-risk zone resides between 40 degrees north and 40 degrees south. Adult immigrants from a high- to a low-risk area carry some of their increased risk with them but infants and young children do not.

All attempts to isolate a viral, spirochetal, or bacterial transmissible agent have been negative to date. Studies of antibody titers to known viruses have shown that anti-measles titers are statistically higher in patients with multiple sclerosis than in the general population.

No important racial, climatic, atmospheric, toxic, or dietary factors have been established in spite of intensive study, nor have factors such as pregnancy, trauma, and intercurrent infection been definitely shown to precipitate relapses. Although the incidence of the disease is 8 times greater in immediate relatives of patients with the disease than in the general population, this does not necessarily indicate an inherited factor, but could reflect a common exposure as is the case in poliomyelitis, where there is a similar increased incidence among relatives.

The inflammatory nature of early lesions, the demonstration of antimyelin antibodies in blood and cerebrospinal fluid, and the tendency to a relapsing clinical course, along with certain pathologic similarities to experimental allergic encephalomyelitis, have suggested the possibility of an auto-immune pathogenetic mechanism involving a component of myelin. However, it must be remembered that auto-immunity can occur as a consequence of certain infections.

There is no evidence that uninvolved myelin in patients with multiple sclerosis differs from that of normals. Myelin breakdown products in the involved areas do not differ in any way from those of other types of destructive lesions. There is no suggestion of any specific aberration of lipid synthesis or catabolism.

Pathologic Features

The characteristic lesion of multiple sclerosis is the "plaque," a sharply localized, irregularly shaped area of discoloration, usually about 0.5 to 2.0 cm in diameter although occasionally larger (Figs. 6.1, 6.2). A recent plaque is yellowish-white or pink as a result of fatty break-down products and congestion; old plaques are translucent, gray-brown, and somewhat firmer in consistency than surrounding tissues. Plaques

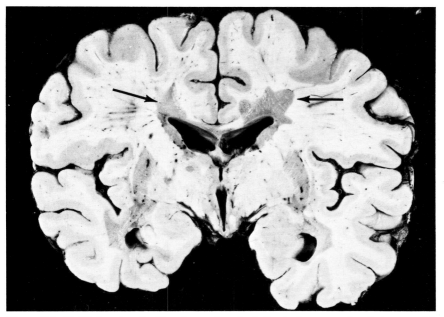

Figure 6.1. Multiple sclerosis. Two large, sharply defined plaques are located symmetri-cally at the angles of the bodies of the lateral ventricles, involving the adjacent white mat-ter and corpus callosum (*arrows*). Other plaques are seen adjacent to the inferior horns and in the thalamus and globus pallidus on the *left*.

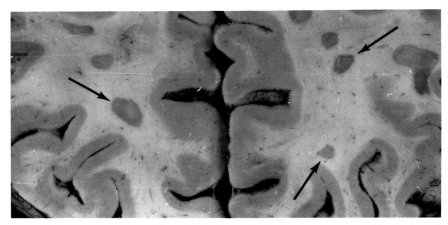

Figure 6.2. Multiple sclerosis. Several sharply outlined plaques are scattered in the frontal white matter (*arrows*).

of different ages are frequently seen to co-exist, corresponding to the multiple clinical episodes.

In acute plaques, the outstanding histologic features are the breakdown of myelin sheaths and reduction or complete loss of the interfascicular oligodendroglia. Large numbers of macrophages contain phagocytosed myelin in various stages of digestion (Fig. 6.3). Lymphocytes and mononuclear cells accumulate in perivascular spaces and in adjacent meninges (Fig. 6.4). Axons are often irregularly swollen or beaded and there may be some fragmentation, but generally most axons persist. As the plaque matures, macrophages become fewer in number and astrocytes proliferate to form a glial scar ("sclerosis"). Old plaques appear as sharply outlined areas of demyelination and dense gliosis (Fig. 6.5) with relatively intact axons (Fig. 6.6). Neuronal cell bodies included in plaques (as in the pons) are also largely spared. Occasionally, however, necrotizing lesions leave reticulated or cystic areas; conversely, incomplete demyelination leads to formation of "shadow plaques."

Plaques are found throughout the central nervous system, and consequently almost any focal neurologic sign may be found in multiple sclerosis. The optic nerves, the tegmentum of the brainstem (Fig. 6.7), cerebellar peduncles, and spinal cord are the most commonly affected areas. In the cerebrum, plaques are most often near the angles of the lateral ventricles or close to the junction of cortex with white matter, and tend to be symmetrically located.

Clinical Findings

The clinical picture will depend upon the location and size of plaques although the pathologic changes are generally more widespread than suggested by the clinical findings. In the early stages, signs are those of one or more acute focal lesions anywhere in the central nervous system. Symptoms usually develop rapidly over 1 or 2 days, but this is often followed by marked improvement, with little functional deficit remaining after a few weeks when axonal conduction is restored. Ninety percent of patients have a relapsing and remitting course in the early stages, but accumulated incomplete recovery leads to a gradual increase in permanent disability. Younger patients occasionally experience a severe fulminating illness from the outset, whereas onset in middle age is usually associated with a more indolent course. Contrary to common belief, one-third of patients run a rather benign course without serious disability or reduction of their life span.

Evidence of spinal cord damage (weakness or numbness in one or more extremities) and monocular blindness or scotoma due to involve-

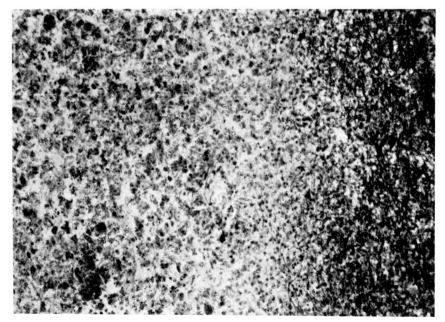

Figure 6.3. Multiple sclerosis. A recent plaque shows loss of myelin sheaths and numerous lipid-containing macrophages. Uninvolved sheaths are seen on the *right*. (Oil red O-iron hematoxylin, × 125)

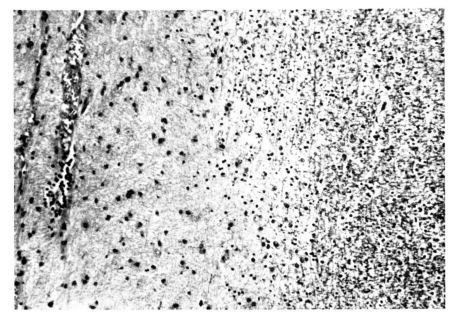

Figure 6.4. Multiple sclerosis. A plaque occupies the *left half* of the photograph. A few lymphocytes occupy a perivascular space. Astrocytes exhibit moderate hypertrophy; oligodendroglial nuclei are markedly reduced in number. Edema is present in the adjacent white matter. (Hematoxylin-phloxine-saffron, × 125)

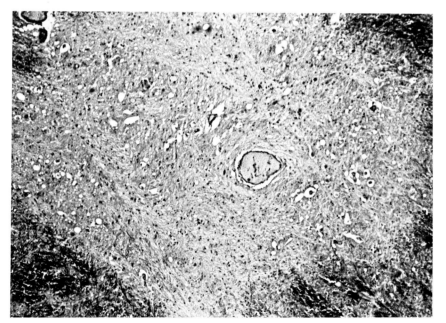

Figure 6.5. Multiple sclerosis. An old perivascular plaque is delineated sharply from adjacent white matter. (Luxol fast blue-hematoxylin-eosin (LFB-HE), × 45)

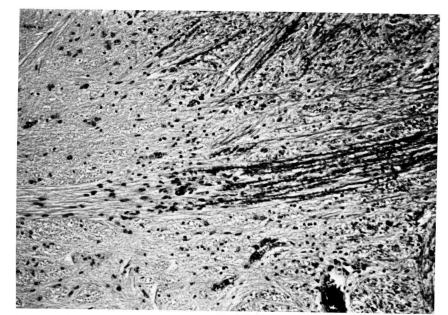

Figure 6.6. Multiple sclerosis. Horizontally placed bundles of axons lose their myelin sheaths at the edge of a plaque, but the axons are intact. (Luxol fast blue-Bodian, × 125)

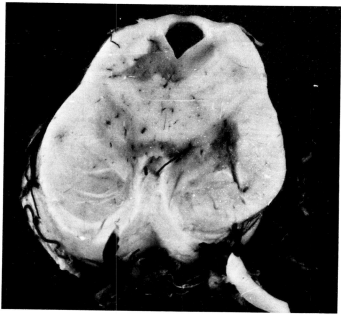

Figure 6.7. Multiple sclerosis. High pons. Plaques occupy periventricular tegmentum and base.

ment of the optic nerve, are common first symptoms. Spastic weakness, nystagmus, pathologic deep and superficial reflexes, cerebellar incoordination, and disturbance of posterior column sensation are frequent physical findings. In the early stages, abnormal physical signs are often more frequent than would be anticipated from the history, the patient being unaware of a minor defect. Pyramidal and cerebellar signs are less likely to improve with time than are visual or sensory defects.

In those patients in whom the disease is progressive, spastic paraplegia leads eventually to confinement in bed and, when associated with incontinence of bladder or bowel, presents a major problem in nursing. Intercurrent infections accentuate any neurologic disability, especially the spastic weakness and associated flexor spasms. Problems in care may be complicated by changes in mental state including intellectual deterioration, euphoria, or depressive reactions.

There are no laboratory tests diagnostic of multiple sclerosis. The total protein content of the cerebrospinal fluid is usually normal or only slightly elevated. However, the globulin component of the cerebrospinal fluid protein is elevated in two-thirds of patients and is presumably produced by cells in the inflammatory lesions. Although no conclusive observations are available concerning the nature of the newly-formed globulin, there has been much interest in a possible immune myelinolytic action or in its role as an antibody to viruses. A mild mononuclear pleocytosis of the cerebrospinal fluid may be found during acute attacks.

Variations of Multiple Sclerosis

In Devic's syndrome (neuromyelitis optica), the lesions predominantly involve the optic pathways and the spinal cord. The onset is acute with serious initial disability. In the majority of patients the spinal cord plaques are large, extending over many segments and showing considerable necrosis as well as demyelination, but other lesions more characteristic of multiple sclerosis are usually found in other parts of the nervous system. In a few instances where progression to death is rapid, the lesions more closely resemble those of acute disseminated encephalomyelitis.

The obsolete terms "Schilder's disease" or "diffuse cerebral sclerosis" may be applied to an uncommon, severe variant of multiple sclerosis occurring most often in adolescents and young adults. Very large confluent plaques occupy much of the white matter of the cerebral hemispheres, and smaller lesions resembling those of multiple sclerosis are seen elsewhere. Unfortunately, these terms are also used to encompass certain childhood familial disorders affecting white matter (leukodystrophies) which are clearly unrelated to multiple sclerosis. According to Lumsden, Schilder described three cases of "diffuse cerebral sclerosis," one probably related to multiple sclerosis, one a familial leukodystrophy, and the third, most likely an adult subacute sclerosing panencephalitis. The feature common to all was, of course, widespread destruction and gliosis of the white matter.

In the usual case of multiple sclerosis coming to autopsy after an illness of 10 to 25 years, most plaques are old and inactive, and it is difficult to find one with active inflammatory changes and myelin breakdown. Occasionally the disease appears to be slowly but continuously active at the margin of the lesions, and this may explain the slowly progressive deterioration seen in some patients, especially the middle-aged.

Of particular interest are those few patients who many years previously have had evidence of one or two discrete lesions (for example, transient monocular blindness), who subsequently remain well and at autopsy years later are shown to have one or two plaques. It would be important to know what factors have prevented the usual evolution of the disease.

ACUTE DISSEMINATED ENCEPHALOMYELITIS

Acute disseminated encephalomyelitis is a relatively rare complication of a number of viral diseases (measles, chickenpox, smallpox, upper respiratory infections, etc.) and some vaccinations, for example smallpox and rabies. The incidence varies widely in different series from 1 in 100,000 to 40 in 100,000 following smallpox vaccination and perhaps 1 in 1,000 following measles infection. Occasional cases occur in the absence of a clearly defined antecedent infection. Most cases occur in children and young adults; it is rare before 2 years of age.

The neurologic illness develops about 5 to 15 days after the onset of the initial infection, with evidence of meningeal irritation, convulsions, confusion, somnolence, and a variety of focal signs referable to apparently random lesions of the cerebrum, brainstem, and spinal cord, any of which may dominate the clinical picture.

The morphologic changes are similar regardless of the antecedent disease. There are usually no distinctive gross changes, although in fulminant cases, scattered petechial hemorrhages are found in white matter. The histologic lesions occur in any myelinated portion of the nervous system, notably in the centrum semiovale and base of the pons, and consist of innumerable tiny foci of perivenular demyelination infiltrated by lymphocytes and macrophages (Figs. 6.8, 6.9). Vascular ne-

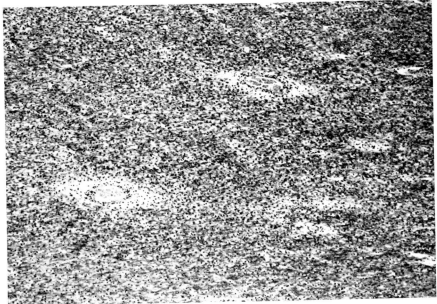

Figure 6.8. Acute disseminated encephalomyelitis. There are multiple scattered small foci of perivascular demyelination and cellular infiltration. (LFB-HE, × 45)

crosis and perivascular hemorrhages are occasionally present. Large lesions produced by confluence of foci may closely resemble plaques of acute multiple sclerosis.

The lesions of disseminated encephalomyelitis are very similar regardless of the nature of the antecedent illness and closely resemble the lesions of experimental allergic encephalitis (*vide infra*). The pathologic appearance and the failure to isolate a virus from the lesions suggest that an auto-immune process is involved, although the immunologic data required to confirm this hypothesis are not yet available.

PARAINFECTIOUS NEURITIS

Lesions of demyelination and inflammation similar to those found in the central nervous system in disseminated encephalomyelitis may also be found in the peripheral nerves, particularly the nerve roots, either in association with disseminated encephalomyelitis (notably following rabies vaccination), or as isolated mono- or polyneuropathies with little or no involvement of brain and spinal cord. The latter are often associated with mild respiratory infections, presumably viral in nature. Again, the pathology is basically that of demyelination with variable but often minimal axonal loss.

THE LANDRY-GUILLAIN-BARRÉ SYNDROME

The Landry-Guillain-Barré syndrome of acute "infectious" polyneuritis is considered by many to be a primary demyelinating disease. It frequently occurs in relation to minor viral infections, and may be found in association with infectious mononucleosis. Involvement is predominantly of nerve roots and proximal nerves (Figs. 6.10, 6.11). Longer axons may be affected first, producing the clinical picture of ascending flaccid paralysis, but sometimes the weakness affects all four limbs simultaneously. Motor cranial nerves and the muscles of respiration are often involved. Sensory changes are mild in comparison to the motor deficit. Sphincters are involved infrequently. On rare occasions the disease adopts a relapsing and remitting course. When inflammation involves the intra-arachnoidal portions of the nerve roots, protein-rich edema fluid escapes from the lesions to produce a marked elevation of cerebrospinal fluid protein out of proportion to the slight pleocytosis—so-called "albuminocytologic dissociation."

Ultrastructural studies have provided support for the hypothesis that there is primary demyelination of the type seen in experimental allergic encephalomyelitis and experimental allergic neuropathy. In addition,

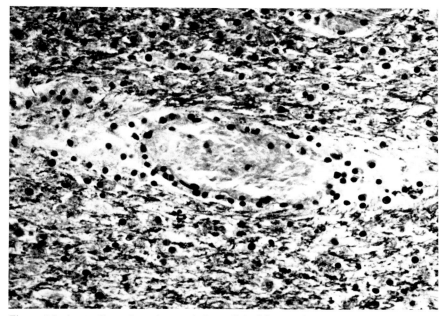

Figure 6.9. Acute disseminated encephalomyelitis. Mononuclear cells infiltrate the perivascular white matter. Myelin sheaths show irregularities and fragmentation. (LFB-HE, × 300)

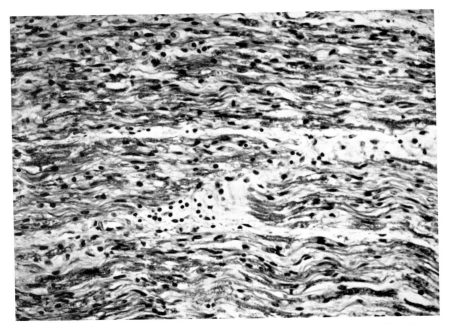

Figure 6.10. Acute infectious polyneuritis. Edema and mononuclear infiltration of proximal portion of a spinal nerve. There is early myelin breakdown and phagocytosis near the *top* of the photograph. (LFB-HE, × 125)

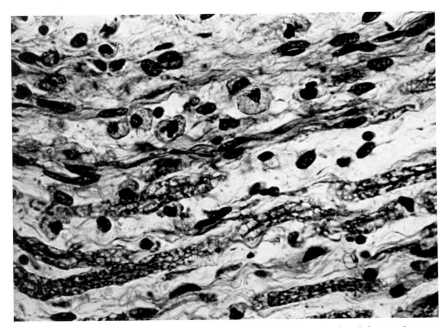

Figure 6.11. Acute infectious polyneuritis. Marked edema, myelin breakdown, phagocytosis, and cellular infiltration in a nerve root. (LFB-HE, × 300)

a complement-dependent serum factor capable of demyelinating peripheral nerve tissue cultures has recently been demonstrated in several cases.

Because necrosis and axonal loss are often minimal, the patient who survives the acute illness generally experiences quite good return of function over several weeks or months. If death occurs in the acute phase, it is usually the result of respiratory failure or infection. Therefore, very careful nursing is required during that period. This is best done in special units having adequate facilities for monitoring blood gases and electrolytes, airway function, and nutrition.

Whether or not they are evoked by infection, the demyelinating diseases appear to involve activation of the immune response. Accordingly, the therapeutic usefulness of immunosuppressive drugs is now being assessed. Corticosteroids are often used, although their benefit remains uncertain.

EXPERIMENTAL AUTO-IMMUNE (ALLERGIC) ENCEPHALOMYELITIS

The occasional occurrence in humans of paralysis following a course of Pasteur rabies vaccine (an emulsion of rabbit brain containing attenuated virus) suggested that injection of extracts of nervous tissue could be damaging to the nervous system of the recipient. This was confirmed by Rivers and co-workers during the 1930's. Monkeys with repeated intradermal injections of an emulsion of brain tissue developed disseminated encephalomyelitis resembling post-vaccinal encephalomyelitis in humans.

In subsequent years, a single injection of brain emulsion with Freund's or other adjuvant was found to produce a high yield of disseminated encephalomyelitis in most of the species tested. The role of the immune mechanism in this disease was widely accepted and the term experimental allergic encephalomyelitis came into general use. Experimental allergic encephalomyelitis has been the subject of numerous investigations both as a model of auto-immune disease and because of its possible relevance to demyelinating diseases in humans, although the latter point has been the subject of much debate.

The principal encephalitogenic antigen is a component of normal myelin sheaths, and is a basic protein located in the intraperiod line in the lamellar structure of myelin. The encephalitogenic determinant is a short peptide of known sequence. Heterologous, isologous, or autologous nervous tissue will induce experimental allergic encephalomyelitis in susceptible animals.

Following injection, both circulating antibodies and a cell-mediated immune response are induced. Attempts to transfer the disease passively to non-immunized allogenic animals using serum have been unsuccessful, whereas transfer of lymphoid cells will usually induce the disease within 3 to 5 days. Although this suggests that the principal mechanism in experimental allergic encephalomyelitis is delayed (tuberculin-type) hypersensitivity, a role for 7S cytotoxic antibodies is by no means eliminated; the latter are capable in brain tissue cultures of producing dissolution of myelin sheaths and degeneration of glial elements, and they do appear in the serum of rats which have received sensitized lymphoid cells in passive transfer experiments.

Experimental allergic encephalomyelitis begins about 10 to 12 days after immunizing injection. Various species and strains of experimental animals exhibit marked differences in severity and duration of the disease. The lesions are largely confined to white matter, and consist of numerous minute foci of perivenous cellular infiltration (largely mononuclear cells), with swelling and fragmentation of myelin sheaths, occasionally progressing to frank necrosis of all tissue elements. In general, axons tend to be spared in mild lesions, in contrast to the conspicuous damage to myelin sheaths. There may also be an associated vasculitis with focal hemorrhages.

Mononuclear cells appear to produce demyelination by directly attacking and disrupting the myelin sheaths and oligodendroglial cells, suggesting that they are sensitized to some element in the membranes. As well, exudation of plasma proteins through abnormally permeable capillaries may bring circulating cytotoxic antibodies into the area.

Injections of peripheral nerve rather than central nervous system tissue produces, in some species, acute demyelination and inflammation of peripheral nerves, most notably the proximal portions. The morphologic and immunologic features are essentially identical with those of experimental allergic encephalomyelitis.

There is thus considerable evidence to support the view that primary demyelination can occur on the basis of immune injury. It seems reasonable to suspect that post-rabies vaccine encephalomyelitis is of the same nature when vaccines containing emulsified brain have been used. The parainfectious demyelinating diseases may be a reflection of interactive antigenicity between virus proteins and myelin sheaths. The role of the immune reaction in multiple sclerosis is, however, uncertain but is under active investigation by several groups. It must be emphasized that the lesions of multiple sclerosis differ in many ways from those of experimental allergic encephalomyelitis and attempts to produce a chronic, relapsing form of experimental allergic encephalomyelitis have thus far been unsuccessful.

REFERENCES

BALDWIN, G. S., AND CARNEGIE, P. R. Specific enzymic methylation of an arginine in the experimental allergic encephalomyelitis protein from human myelin. Science 171:579, 1971.

BORNSTEIN, M. B., AND IWANAMI, H. Experimental allergic encephalomyelitis: demyelinating activity of serum and sensitized lymph node cells on cultured nerve tissues. J. Neuropath. Exp. Neurol. 30:240, 1971.

DOWLING, P. C., AND COOK, S. D. Pattern of cellular and humoral events in experimental allergic encephalomyelitis. Neurology (Minneap.) 18:953, 1968.

HIRANO, A., COOK, S. D., WHITAKER, J. N., DOWLING, P. C., AND MURRAY, M. R. Fine structural aspects of demyelination in vitro. The effects of Guillain-Barré serum. J. Neuropath. Exp. Neurol. 30:249, 1971.

KIM, S. U., MURRAY, M. R., TOURTELLOTTE, W. W., AND PARKER, J. A. Demonstration in tissue culture of myelinotoxicity in cerebrospinal fluid and brain extracts from multiple sclerosis patients. J. Neuropath. Exp. Neurol. 29:420, 1970.

KURTZKE, J. F., BEEBE, G. W., NAGLER, B., NEFZGER, M. D., AUTH, T. L., AND KURLAND, L. T. Studies on natural history of multiple sclerosis: V. Long-term survival in young men. Arch. Neurol. (Chicago) 22:215, 1970.

MATTHEWS, W. B., HOWELL, D. A., AND HUGHES, R. C. Relapsing corticosteroid-dependent polyneuritis. J. Neurol. Neurosurg. Psychiat. 33:330, 1970.

PATERSON, P. Y. Experimental autoimmune (allergic) encephalomyelitis. *In* Textbook of Immunopathology. Ed. by P. A. Miescher and H. J. Muller-Eberhard. Grune & Stratton, Inc., New York and London, 1968.

SPILLANE, J. D., AND WELLS, C. E. C. The neurology of Jennerian vaccination. Brain 87:1, 1964.

SUZUKI, K., ASBURY, A. K., ARNASON, B. G., AND ADAMS, R. D. The inflammatory lesion in idiopathic polyneuritis: its role in pathogenesis. Medicine (Balt.) 48:173, 1969.

SUZUKI, K., ANDREWS, J. M., WALTZ, J. M., AND TERRY, R. D. Ultrastructural studies of multiple sclerosis. Lab. Invest. 20:444, 1969.

WEIDERHOLDT, W., MULDER, D., AND LAMBERT, E. The Landry-Guillain-Barré-Strohl syndrome of polyradiculoneuropathy. Historical review, report on 97 patients, and present concepts. Mayo Clin. Proc. 39:427, 1964.

7

INFECTIOUS DISEASES

INTRODUCTION

The central nervous system is well protected from microbiologic agents by its coverings and by the body's defense mechanisms. However, nearly all pathogenetic bacteria, viruses, fungi, treponemas, rickettsiae, and protozoa may gain entry to the nervous system, and when immune resources are depressed, organisms which as a rule are non-pathogenetic in man may produce serious disease.

Routes and Predisposing Factors

Most central nervous system infections are blood-borne, having been carried from foci elsewhere in the body. The neurologic involvement may be a complication of an inconspicuous primary infection, such as a mild pharyngitis, or arise from a clinically apparent pneumonia, endocarditis, or other infection. The host factors determining dissemination in individual cases are usually obscure. In general, the most susceptible are the very young and very old, debilitated patients, diabetics, and patients with disorders of immunologic mechanisms. A number of neurologic diseases proven or thought to be infectious, such as progressive multifocal leukoencephalopathy, occur most often as late complications of lymphomas, leukemias, and carcinomas.

Direct implantation of organisms occurs as a result of penetrating wounds of the skull or spinal canal. Basal skull fractures may disrupt the dura and the mucosa of the nasopharynx and external auditory canal, permitting entry of bacteria, notably pneumococci and staphylococci. Infections may also spread through bone or along venous channels (thrombophlebitis) from foci in the face, scalp, paranasal sinuses, middle ears, and mastoid air cells. Children with chronic bacterial upper respiratory infections or otitis media are prone to intracranial infections.

Effects of Infections in the Central Nervous System

A prodromal period of vague ill health may precede by a number of days the appearance of symptoms and signs of central nervous system infection. In some of the milder viral illnesses, transient disturbances in neural function result in mild drowsiness and increased irritability, but full recovery is the rule. Other patients pass through a stage of delirium to drowsiness, stupor, and coma. Inflammation of the meninges leads to signs of meningeal irritation, including cervical rigidity with spasm of the extensor muscles of the neck causing head retraction, and pain when passive extension of the knee is attempted with the hip fully flexed (Kernig's sign). The patient tends to lie in an attitude of mild flexion, is irritable and prefers subdued light or darkness. The deep tendon and superficial cutaneous reflexes may be depressed. Edema of the brain, exudation, and obstruction of cerebrospinal fluid pathways lead to evidence of increased intracranial pressure, including headache (which may be severe), nausea, vomiting, and papilledema. Various cranial nerve palsies may result from direct infiltration of the nerves by the inflammatory process or as a result of compression from cerebral swelling. Focal damage to the cerebral hemispheres may cause epileptic convulsions which may recur as a chronic complication, particularly in children. In the more protracted subacute infections, an infectious arteritis or thrombophlebitis may occur in cerebral vessels and cause cerebral ischemia or frank infarction. Occasionally, patients who have made a recovery satisfactory in most respects are left with a mild change in personality or a permanent defect in learning ability.

Cerebrospinal Fluid Changes

The diagnostic importance of cerebrospinal fluid examination in infectious diseases cannot be overemphasized. With acute infections of the central nervous system the cerebrospinal fluid is usually under increased pressure. Its appearance will depend upon the number of leukocytes present and ranges from slight turbidity to frank purulence. In the majority of bacterial infections there is a prompt rise in leukocytes, mostly neutrophils, to very high levels. Viral, rickettsial, and mycotic infections are characterized by a preponderance of mononuclear cells, although neutrophils appear in the early stages and in response to massive tissue destruction as seen in Herpes simplex encephalitis. Generally, bacterial infections have much higher cell counts than the viral infections.

On occasion, diffuse infiltration of the meninges by neoplastic cells produces the clinical picture of a meningitis, usually associated with a great deal of nerve root pain. In these patients, cytologic studies for malignant cells in the cerebrospinal fluid may assist diagnosis.

Proteins, largely derived from the plasma, are elevated as a result of increased vascular permeability; occasionally, as with tuberculous meningitis, the fibrinogen content may be so high as to permit a fine coagulum to form if the fluid is left standing. Glucose is reduced in bacterial infections, occasionally to undetectable levels. The cause of the hypoglycorrhachia is not fully understood, but glucose may be metabolized by organisms and inflammatory cells or there may be interference with its transport into the cerebrospinal fluid.

While the cellular and biochemical changes provide some suggestion as to the nature of the infection, the most important step is the identification of the causative organisms by direct smear, culture, and immunologic techniques. This allows institution of rational therapy based on the organisms' proven susceptibility to specific antibiotics or other drugs. Unfortunately, the techniques now generally available for virus identification are too slow to be of much clinical value except in the investigation and control of epidemics. A notable exception is Herpes simplex, which is occasionally found in the cellular sediment using immunofluorescence or electron microscopy.

In view of the very wide range of possible infecting organisms, the microbiologic techniques applied to the individual sample of cerebrospinal fluid must be carefully chosen. Adequate communication between clinician and laboratory physician is essential.

INFECTIONS WITH PYOGENIC BACTERIA

Infections may occur in any of the meningeal compartments—the epidural, subdural, and subarachnoid spaces—or within the substance of the brain or spinal cord. The barriers between compartments tend to limit the spread of infection although they fail to do so in many cases.

Epidural and Subdural Abscesses

Epidural and subdural infections usually follow penetrating head injuries or extension of infection from adjacent bone and paranasal sinuses. Intracranial epidural abscesses are generally well localized because of the adherence of the dura to the inner table of the skull, but spinal epidural infections spread through the epidural fat and venous plexus. Subdural abscesses spread widely through the subdural space, become loculated by fibrinous and fibrous adhesions, are much more difficult to drain surgically, and carry a higher mortality. Both types show the usual gross and histologic features of acute purulent inflammation, and in time incite fibrosis in the adjacent tissues. Their effects on adjacent brain or spinal cord are predominantly those of compression although there may be direct extension of the infection to these structures.

Leptomeningitis

The majority of pyogenic infections of the nervous system are hematogenous in origin and involve the subarachnoid space. Among the organisms commonly implicated are Escherichia coli and Haemophilus influenzae in infants and children, and Streptococcus pneumoniae in older adults. Neisseria meningitidis has produced occasional outbreaks in military camps and boarding schools where close proximity of individuals favors direct spread of the organism. Many other bacteria may produce leptomeningitis, and their identification is essential for the judicious selection of antibiotic therapy. The widespread use of antibiotics has resulted in the appearance of drug-resistant strains and a change in the prevalence of some organisms. For example, Staphylococcus aureus has been responsible for a larger percentage of cases of meningitis in adults in recent years.

Appearance

In the acute stage the organisms and exudate become widely disseminated throughout the subarachnoid space and frequently involve the ventricular cavities (Fig. 7.1.). The exudate, composed predominantly of neutrophils (Fig. 7.2), produces opacity of the subarachnoid space, obscuring anatomic markings and vessels over the surface of the brain, a feature particularly evident in the major sulci. Shaggy masses of pus may coat the choroid plexuses and ependymal surfaces with cranial and spinal nerves encased and infiltrated by the exudate. After a few days, increasing numbers of macrophages, lymphocytes, and plasma cells appear and deposits of fibrin are seen (Fig. 7.3). Fibroblastic proliferation is a variable feature, and occurs after 1 or 2 weeks.

Infection frequently spreads into cerebral perivascular spaces, but the pial-glial barrier is remarkably effective in preventing extension to the neural parenchyma. Occasionally, however, multiple focal intracerebral abscesses are found.

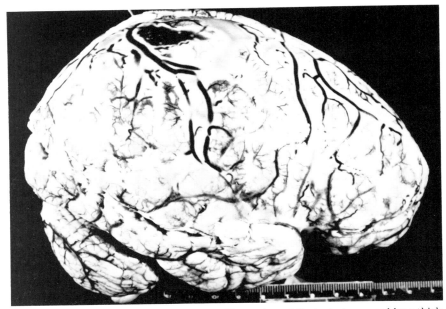

Figure 7.1. Acute bacterial leptomeningitis. The surface of the brain is covered by a thick purulent exudate which obscures the normal anatomic markings. Surface veins have undergone thrombosis.

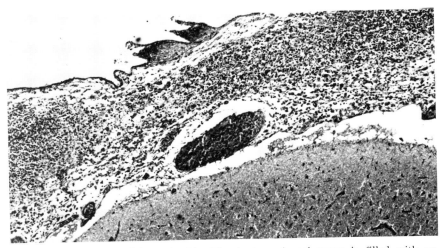

Figure 7.2. Acute bacterial meningitis. The leptomeningeal space is filled with an exudate which at higher power was composed largely of neutrophils. The pial surface (*below*) and the outer arachnoid membrane (*above*) delimit spread of the infection. (Hematoxylin-eosin (HE), × 60)

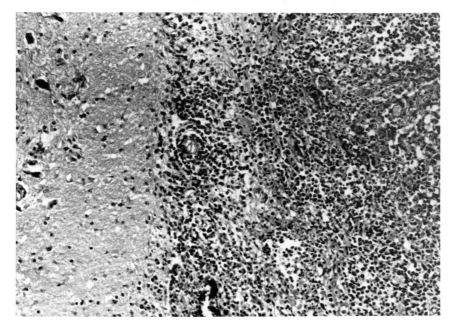

Figure 7.3. Acute leptomeningitis, resolving. In addition to neutrophils, the exudate contains many mononuclear cells. Much fibrin is present. (HE, × 125)

Complications

Prompt and vigorous therapy in the initial stages in an otherwise healthy patient usually results in resolution of the infection with little or no residual damage.

In the acute phase, septic thrombophlebitis of surface veins or the major sinuses may produce hemorrhagic infarction. The exudate occasionally blocks cerebrospinal fluid drainage, producing rapidly progressive hydrocephalus.

The major late complication is obstructive hydrocephalus which is the result of meningeal fibrosis and usually follows delayed or inadequate therapy of the acute illness.

Cerebral Abscess

Microorganisms may reach the substance of the brain by implantation or direct extension from neighboring structures, but hematogenous spread is the most frequent route. Chronic bronchopulmonary, paranasal sinus, and middle ear infections and congenital heart lesions with right to left shunting and endocarditis are frequent sources.

Appearance

Brain abscesses may be in any location but are usually near the source if local spread is involved. Hematogenous spread frequently leads to multiple abscesses which appear to develop near the junction of cortex and white matter.

The initial reaction is said to be a focal "cerebritis" which subsequently liquefies to form an abscess cavity (Fig. 7.4). The cavity is filled with purulent exudate and progressively enlarges by destruction of brain tissue at its edges and fusion with adjacent foci. The surrounding brain is very soft and swollen, adding further to the increased intracranial mass. There is proliferation of reactive astrocytes, but these seem ineffective in controlling the progress of the infection and frequently show degenerative changes.

After a few days, proliferation of fibroblasts and small blood vessels occurs at the edges. Gradually, a connective tissue capsule containing macrophages, lymphocytes, and plasma cells is built up around the abscess (Fig. 7.5). Chronic, long-standing abscesses may be walled off

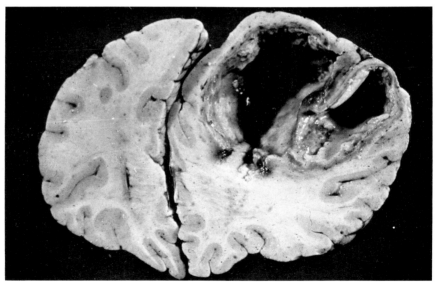

Figure 7.4. Cerebral abscess. A biloculate abscess cavity, the liquid contents removed, occupies much of the frontal white matter. There is also marked cerebral edema and subfalcine shift.

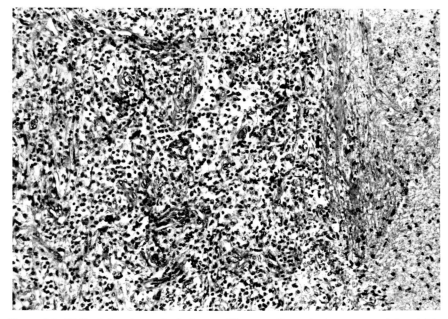

Figure 7.5. Wall of chronic cerebral abscess. The necrotic contents are seen at the *right*. The capsule, occupying the remainder of the photograph, is composed of granulation tissue with leukocytes and mononuclear cells. (HE, × 125)

by the fibrous capsule. It should be noted that this is one of the comparatively few circumstances in which a connective tissue scar, rather than a glial scar, is formed in the central nervous system. The neurosurgeon generally finds that the mature capsule can be separated easily from the surrounding soft, edematous brain tissue.

Complications

The effects of a brain abscess are those of local tissue destruction and irritation and of a rapidly expanding intracranial mass with herniations. Rupture into a ventricle or subarachnoid space produces rapidly progressive leptomeningitis.

Untreated abscesses are usually fatal; however, surgical drainage and antibiotic therapy are highly effective. The residual scarring may act as an epileptogenic focus. In recent years improved antibiotic therapy has resulted in better control of infectious diseases and their complications and the incidence of cerebral abscess has declined markedly. However, the clinician must be constantly on guard not to overlook the possibility of cerebral abscess in a patient with symptoms of a focal and possibly expanding intracranial lesion with a mild pleocytosis and elevated protein in the cerebrospinal fluid.

TUBERCULOSIS

Although once quite common, tuberculosis of the central nervous system has responded well to vigorous public health measures. Infection continues to occur with relatively high frequency in parts of Asia and among the Eskimos and Indians of northern Canada. The central nervous system involvement arises by hematogenous dissemination, usually from a pulmonary focus.

Tuberculous meningitis follows a more protracted course than pyogenic meningitis. Exudate is especially abundant at the base of the brain where it involves the cranial nerves and may produce a granulomatous arteritis with subsequent thrombosis. The histologic features are similar to tuberculosis elsewhere, although the granulomas are often not so discrete as in other organs, and diffuse exudation, fibrin deposition, and necrosis are prominent.

Tuberculomas, or tuberculous abscesses, arise within the brain substance and behave as slowly expanding masses. They consist of a large core of caseous necrosis surrounded by granulomatous inflammation and a fibrous capsule; calcification may occur (Fig. 7.6).

Tuberculous spinal epidural granulomas secondary to vertebral osteomyelitis have become rare indeed.

SARCOIDOSIS

Intracranial sarcoidosis, although not known to be infectious, is conveniently inserted here because it has many features in common with tuberculosis or other chronic infections. It produces a chronic granulomatous basal meningitis which entraps cranial nerves and may destroy structures in the hypothalamus and adjacent to the third ventricle. Occasionally, widespread granulomas occur in the substance of the brain.

Cerebrospinal fluid findings of pleocytosis, high protein, and decreased glucose are highly suggestive of infection but attempts to identify organisms fail. Biopsy of lymph nodes, other involved organs, or meninges may be required for diagnosis, particularly when the systemic features of sarcoidosis are minimal or absent.

FUNGAL INFECTIONS

A very large number of fungi have been implicated as causes of neurologic infection and their frequency is said to have increased in

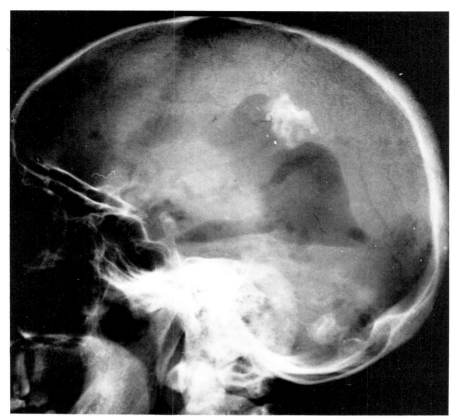

Figure 7.6. Tuberculosis. X-rays of a 44 year old Eskimo with seizures and right hemiparesis. Calcification of tuberculomas in left cerebral hemisphere and cerebellum. Pneumoencephalogram shows dilated left lateral ventricle.

recent years. Most fungal infections are associated with malnutrition, diabetes, lymphomas, carcinomas, or other states in which host resistance is impaired. Instances have been reported following organ transplantation and immunosuppressive therapy. There are reports of fungal infection following parenteral self-administration of narcotics. Occasionally, no predisposing factors can be identified.

Spread to the nervous system is almost always hematogenous, from foci in the lungs or elsewhere, although the primary focus may be inconspicuous. The meninges or neural parenchyma, or both, may be involved. Gross and microscopic appearances vary widely but in general there is slowly progressive purulent or granulomatous meningitis

(Fig. 7.7) or formation of chronic brain abscesses, and a marked tendency to obliterative meningeal fibrosis.

Diagnosis rests principally on identification of the causative fungus in cerebrospinal fluid or tissue specimens or on appropriate immunologic procedures. Although treatment is very difficult and mortality is extremely high, some agents have proven to be therapeutically effective. Therefore, one should persist in attempting to identify an organism from repeated cerebrospinal fluid examination.

VIRAL DISEASES

The acute viral encephalitides have been well known for many years. One of the truly significant advances in the neurosciences in recent years, however, has been the demonstration that the brain may react to virus infections other than by acute inflammation; in fact, inflammation—a hallmark of the acute viral infections—may be absent.

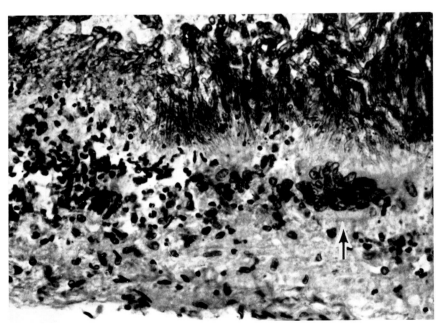

Figure 7.7 Fungal meningitis. A colony of branching hyphae (Aspergillus) has resulted in granulomatous meningitis with giant cells (*arrow*) and evidence of recent necrosis. (Hematoxylin-van Gieson, × 325)

Virus-Induced Malformations

It has been shown convincingly that maternal rubella infection acquired during the first 10 to 12 weeks of pregnancy may pass the placental barrier, infect the fetus, and produce a high incidence of fetal malformations involving the brain, ear, eye, heart, and other organs. The virus commonly persists in the infant's tissues for several months after birth. In the brain, the usual finding is microcephaly with associated mental retardation. Microgyria, agenesis of the corpus callosum, and meningomyelocele have been present in some cases. Histologic changes are meager and include patchy gliosis of white matter, and deposits of periodic acid-Schiff-positive material and calcification near vessels in the basal ganglia and elsewhere.

Our understanding of the role of other viruses is incomplete. There is some evidence that mumps, measles, influenza, and infectious hepatitis occurring in early pregnancy are associated with a slightly increased incidence of cerebral malformations.

Experimental models have been valuable in helping to explain the mechanisms involved. Newborn hamsters injected intracerebrally with mumps virus appear clinically normal, but the virus infects and destroys ependymal cells, producing extensive ulceration of the ventricular surfaces and a mild inflammatory reaction. No virus is detected after 9 days. During the next several weeks, 95 percent of animals develop stenosis or occlusion of the aqueduct of Sylvius and obstructive hydrocephalus. Neither inflammation nor evidence of viral activity is present at the time hydrocephalus occurs.

Margolis, Kilham, and co-workers have demonstrated that several parvoviruses, which have an affinity for rapidly dividing cell populations, are able to destroy the immature external granular layer of the cerebellar cortex when infection occurs in the late fetal or early neonatal stages in a number of species. The cerebellar infection produces a brief phase of intense cellular necrosis that results in profound depletion of the granule cell population—so-called granuloprival cerebellar hypoplasia, closely resembling one form of cerebellar hypoplasia seen in humans.

Acute Viral Encephalomyelitis

Three principal routes of spread of viruses to the nervous system are known of which the most important is the hematogenous. Virus multiplication occurs first at the initial point of entry, such as the gastrointestinal mucosa in poliomyelitis, or the subcutaneous tissue and vascular endothelium at the site of an insect bite in arbovirus infections. The viruses later enter the blood, cross the vascular barrier into the brain, possibly by endothelial pinocytosis, and replicate in neural or glial cells.

Rabies virus reaches the central nervous system via the peripheral nerves located at the site of infection, by a process that involves both replication and extracellular diffusion. Herpes simplex may on occasion enter the brain through the olfactory mucosa, a mechanism that might explain its predominant localization in the orbital and medial temporal areas; however, hematogenous dissemination appears the rule.

Appearances

In most viral infections neurons are severely and predominantly affected. They undergo necrosis, stimulating a cellular response in which a few neutrophils and later macrophages participate (neuronophagia) (Fig. 7.8). Some viruses selectively involve certain neuronal groups; the predilection of poliomyelitis for motor neurons in spinal cord and brainstem and of Herpes zoster for dorsal root ganglia are two out-

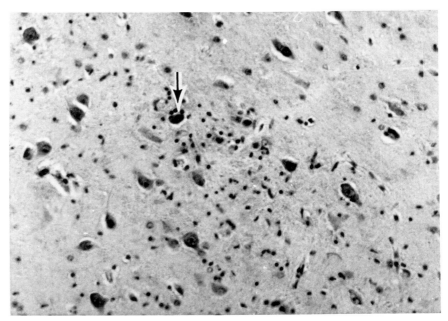

Figure 7.8. Viral meningitis. Hippocampus, showing early lesion with activation of macrophages and evidence of recent neuronal death (*arrow*). (HE, × 125)

standing examples. The majority, however, have inconstant or over-lapping patterns of distribution which are of limited help in histologic diagnosis. The infected neurons may contain cytoplasmic or nuclear inclusion bodies characteristic of the virus involved.

The extent of tissue necrosis varies greatly. In Herpes simplex and several of the arboviruses, large areas of pan-necrosis involve not only neurons, but also glial elements, myelinated fibers, axons, and blood vessels (Fig. 7.9.). Large areas of necrosis of white matter are particu-larly prominent in Western equine encephalitis. In poliomyelitis and rabies, in contrast, necrosis is usually limited to the involved neurons.

Cellular exudation is usually an outstanding histologic feature. The meninges and Virchow-Robin spaces contain numerous lymphocytes and plasma cells whereas in the neuropil neutrophils, macrophages and hypertrophied microglial rod cells predominate. Clusters of the latter, often near blood vessels, are referred to as "glial stars."

Effects

The effects of virus invasion of the central nervous system will depend in part upon the regions most affected. The term encephalitis refers to disease-producing inflammation of the brain whereas myelitis refers to involvement of the spinal cord. In many patients the terms meningo-encephalitis or encephalomyelitis are appropriate. The term polio-myelitis was used originally to refer to involvement of the gray matter of the spinal cord.

The clinical course will depend in general upon the speed of onset and severity of the disease, but in some cases special features of the pathologic process will produce more or less characteristic symptoms. Confusion, dizziness, headache, and drowsiness are non-localizing fea-tures seen in the majority of acute viral encephalitides. Coma will develop if there is severe involvement of the brainstem either directly by the infection or secondary to brainstem compression from cerebral swelling. Epileptic seizures are particularly common with encephalitis in childhood. Signs of temporal lobe necrosis, such as severe memory disturbance, frequently characterize Herpes simplex infection. Polio-myelitis, now seen rarely, usually presents with a transient phase of systemic symptoms followed by evidence of damage to one or more areas of the central nervous system of which the most frequent is spinal anterior horn cell involvement causing lower motor neuron paralysis.

Complete clinical recovery usually follows mild infections. Subtle changes in personality or more striking disturbances in mentation, such as a lengthy period of retrograde amnesia, may be permanent sequelae

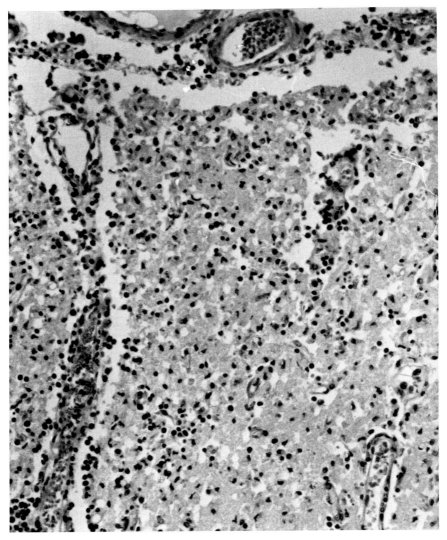

Figure 7.9. Herpes simplex encephalitis. Section of temporal lobe showing massive necrosis of tissue elements, meningeal and perivascular mononuclear infiltration, and numerous macrophages. Neurons and macroglia have been almost totally destroyed. (Hematoxylin-phloxine-saffron, × 350)

of encephalitis. Some infections, including the equine encephalitides, have a propensity for producing permanent intellectual or motor defects in young children but seldom do so in adults.

Slow Virus Infections

In 1954 Sigurdson first used the term "slow infection" to describe such diseases as scrapie and visna, which are chronic neurologic diseases in sheep produced by transmissible agents having most of the properties of viruses. Among the important characteristics were a long latent period of many months or years and a slow, relentlessly progressive clinical course over months or years, ending in death.

Kuru is a slowly progressive fatal disease confined to an isolated mountain tribe in New Guinea where it consituted until recently a major cause of disability and death. Cerebellar ataxia is followed by weakness, dementia, and cranial nerve palsies, and death occurs in a few months or years. Histologically, there is degeneration and loss of neurons and gliosis most evident in the diencephalon, brainstem, and cerebellum, some demyelination of long tracts, and mild cortical degeneration, but little or no inflammatory exudate. The neuronal and other changes have a resemblance to those of scrapie in sheep. Gajdusek and co-workers attempted transmission from fatal human cases to several animal species. After an incubation period of 18 to 30 months, chimpanzees (but not other species) developed a syndrome of ataxia and incoordination which was again transmissible to other chimpanzees. The histologic findings were similar to those in human kuru. Other investigations provided evidence that the familial pattern in human cases was not genetically determined, but was instead the result of a tribal custom of ritualistic cannibalism of the recently deceased by his family, who thus became infected by the agent.

Creutzfeldt-Jakob disease, (subacute spongiform encephalopathy) is a relatively infrequent cause of dementia with extrapyramidal, pyramidal, and occasionally spinal involvement, which usually occurs in middle-aged persons and is fatal in a few months. The changes are those of widespread neuronal degeneration and depletion in cortex, basal ganglia, and elsewhere throughout the neuraxis, with some evidence of phagocytosis and marked astrocytic proliferation. Loss of cortical neurons and marked swelling of remaining neuronal processes often produce a "spongy" appearance of the tissue, hence the term, subacute spongiform encephalopathy, often applied to this condition. Familial cases are the exception. Recently, this disease was also trans-

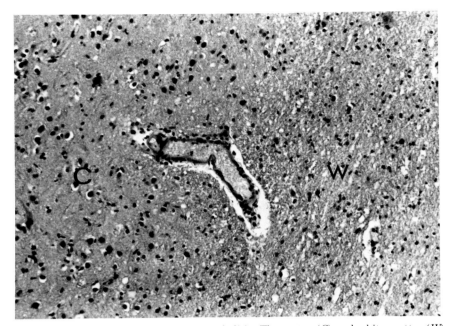

Figure 7.10. Subacute sclerosing panencephalitis. The cortex (*C*) and white matter (*W*) both exhibit evidence of damage and glial proliferation. There is perivascular lymphocytic cuffing. (HE, × 125)

mitted to chimpanzees after a minimum incubation period of 12 months, and thus appears to be another example of a slow virus infection.

Subacute sclerosing panencephalitis is an illness of children and adolescents, the agent of which is a paramyxovirus indistinguishable both morphologically and antigenically from the measles virus. In contrast to the usual systemic measles infection, however, the encephalitis is a slowly progressive illness with widespread neurologic manifestations that result in death after many months or years. The virus attacks both neurons and glia, and produces widespread destruction of both gray and white matter particularly in the cerebral hemispheres (Fig. 7.10). Eosinophilic intranuclear inclusions (Fig. 7.11) composed of tubular myxovirus profiles are found in glial cells.

The majority of patients have a history of measles infection or administration of live measles vaccine, and most have high titers of anti-measles antibody. However, measles is a very common childhood infection and subacute sclerosing panencephalitis is distinctly uncommon; the determinants, whether they reside with the agent or the host, remain to be identified. Recent studies have suggested the simultaneous presence of a second virus.

There are additional entities known or suspected of being slow viral infections, and undoubtedly more will be found. There is at present very active investigation of the possibility that multiple sclerosis and some of the degenerative diseases including motor neuron disease and Parkinson's disease may also be slow infections. The laboratory and animal facilities required for these studies are very costly and the time required is measured in term of many years; these investigations are among the most complex virologic studies yet undertaken.

Remote Effects of Malignant Disease

The association of terminal neoplastic disease, notably the lymphomas, with a variety of infections is well-known. In addition, in recent years a number of neurologic syndromes have been recognized in persons with malignancies not produced by metastases, and occasionally occurring early in the course of the primary disease.

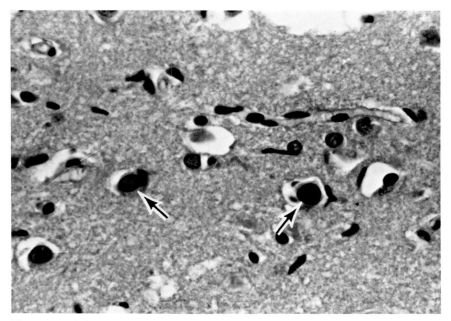

Figure 7.11. Subacute sclerosing panencephalitis. The nuclei of two glial cells (*arrows*) are distended by homogeneous inclusion bodies; chromatin is displaced to the periphery. The inclusions, by electron microscopy, contain paramyxovirus. (HE, × 550)

Progressive multifocal leukoencephalopathy is a low-grade encephalitis which is most often associated with lymphomas, although a few cases have occurred in non-neoplastic circumstances where the immune response is suppressed, for example in the management of patients following renal transplants. There is widespread, patchy destruction of white matter throughout the hemispheres (Fig. 7.12); glial cells undergo marked nuclear enlargement and frequently have intranuclear inclusions which contain papovavirus-like particles.

Subacute cerebellar atrophy is usually associated with carcinoma of the lung, ovary, or gastrointestinal tract and results in progressive cerebellar ataxia. Microscopically, there is widespread destruction of Purkinje cells with gliosis and lymphocytic meningeal infiltration (Fig. 7.13). No causative agent has been identified; however, in some cases there is also evidence of a low-grade encephalitis notably involving brainstem and diencephalon, quite suggestive of a viral etiology.

Other syndromes include sensory and mixed neuropathies, and polymyositis. In elderly individuals, particularly in males, the occurrence of unexplained proximal muscular weakness, wasting, and tenderness may be early evidence of a cryptic malignancy. Whether these are

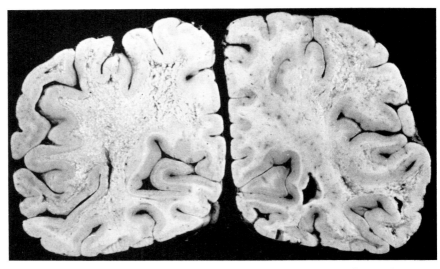

Figure 7.12. Progressive multifocal leukoencephalopathy, following renal transplantation and immunosuppressive therapy. Very severe, widespread necrosis and cavitation of white matter in occipitoparietal region. Papovavirus-like particles were found in glial nuclei by electron microscopy.

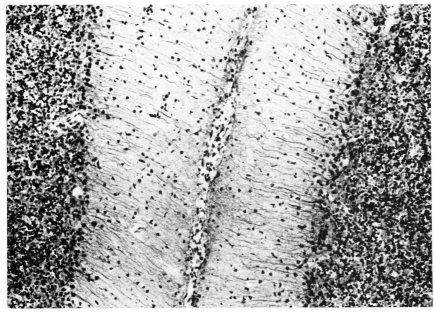

Figure 7.13. Subacute cerebellar atrophy in an elderly man with oat-cell carcinoma of the lung. There is total loss of Purkinje cells, gliosis, and mild lymphocytic infiltration of meninges. (Phosphotungstic acid-hematoxylin, × 130)

also virus infections or some immunologic aberration remains to be determined.

REFERENCES

BRAIN, R., AND NORRIS, F., JR. The Remote Effects of Cancer on the Nervous System. Grune & Stratton, Inc., New York, 1965.

DODGE, P. R., AND SWARTZ, M. N. Bacterial meningitis. II. Special neurologic problems, postmeningitic complications and clinicopathological correlations. New Eng. J. Med. 272:954, 1003, 1965.

DRACHMAN, D. A., AND ADAMS, R. D. Herpes simplex and acute inclusion-body encephalitis. Arch. Neurol. (Chicago) 7:45, 1962.

FETTER, B. F., KLINTWORTH, G. K., AND HENDRY, W. S. Mycoses of the Central Nervous System. The Williams & Wilkins Co., Baltimore, 1967.

GAJDUSEK, D. C., GIBBS, C. J., JR., AND ALPERS, M. Transmission and passage of experimental "kuru" to chimpanzees. Science 155:212, 1967.

GIBBS, C. J., JR., AND GAJDUSEK, D. C. Infection as the etiology of spongiform encephalopathy (Creutzfeldt-Jakob disease). Science 165:1023, 1969.

HOWATSON, A. F., NAGAI, M., AND ZU RHEIN, G. M. Polyoma-like virions in human demyelinating brain disease. Canad. Med. Ass. J. 93:379, 1965.

JOHNSON, R. T., AND JOHNSON, K. P. Hydrocephalus following viral infection: pathology of aqueductal stenosis developing after experimental mumps virus infection. J. Neuropath. Exp. Neurol. 27:591, 1968.

JOHNSON, R. T., AND JOHNSON, K. P. Slow and chronic virus infections of the nervous system. *In* Recent Advances in Neurology. Ed. by F. Plum. F. A. Davis Co., Philadelphia, 1969.

JOHNSON, R. T., AND MIMS, C. A. Pathogenesis of viral infections of the nervous system. New Eng. J. Med. 278:23, 84, 1968.

JONES, H. R., SIEKERT, R. G., AND GERACI, J. E. Neurologic manifestations of bacterial endocarditis. Ann. Intern. Med. 71:21, 1969.

KILHAM, L., MARGOLIS, G., AND COLBY, E. D. Congenital infections of cats and ferrets by feline panleukopenia virus manifested by cerebellar hypoplasia. Lab. Invest. 17:465, 1967.

PAYNE, F. E., BAUBLIS, J. V., AND ITABASHI, H. H. Isolation of measles virus from cell cultures of brain from a patient with subacute sclerosing panencephalitis. New Eng. J. Med. 281:585, 1969.

ROSE, F. C., AND SYMONDS, C. P. Persistent memory defect following encephalitis. Brain 83:195, 1960.

ROZDILSKY, B., ROBERTSON, H. E., AND CHORNEY, J. Western encephalitis: report of eight fatal cases: Saskatchewan epidemic, 1965. Canad. Med. Ass. J. 98:79, 1968.

SWARTZ, M. N., AND DODGE, P. R. Bacterial meningitis. I. General clinical features, special problems and unusual meningeal reactions mimicking bacterial meningitis. New Eng. J. Med. 272:725, 779, 842, 898, 1965.

ZIMMERMAN, H. M. (Ed). Infections of the Nervous System. Association for Research in Nervous and Mental Diseases, Proceedings, Vol. 44. The Williams & Wilkins Co., Baltimore, 1968.

8

TRAUMA

Injuries of the head and spine are medical problems of increasing importance and are very much a part of our civilization. They constitute about 80 percent of injuries and about 70 percent of fatalities in motor vehicle accidents, and among the survivors there may be physical or emotional disturbances that result in lengthy disability and costly litigation. Much has been written on the difficulties inherent in automobile safety engineering; the head and neck are themselves poorly designed to withstand the forces of high energy impacts, and their protection is difficult to achieve.

The vulnerability of the brain to injury in contact sports such as football and hockey is well recognized and helmets and other protective devices are widely used; but unorganized athletic actvities in which supervision and equipment are lacking continue to take their toll. As well, accidents in the home and at work, hunting accidents, and war wounds are major causes of head injury.

HEAD INJURIES

At a gross level, the mechanisms of head injuries are not difficult to understand. The physical force deforms, displaces, and tears the tissues, producing loss of function, necrosis, and hemorrhage in varying degrees of severity and in various combinations. The details, however, are very complex and incompletely understood.

Head injuries may be roughly classified as *closed* where a blunt object damages the brain and its coverings without actually perforating the skull or dura, and *penetrating* when the skull and brain are directly lacerated by an object such as a bullet (Fig. 8.1). The mechanisms involved in the latter type are usually obvious and require no further comment. The closed type, which constitutes the majority of civilian injuries, has a more complicated pathogenesis.

Central to the understanding of the mechanisms of closed head injury is the concept that the brain is a soft, easily deformed mass contained within, but not quite filling, the rigid bony cavity. Thus, when the moving head is abruptly brought to a stop the brain is able to con-

141

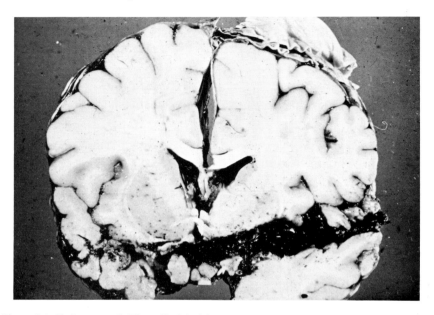

Figure 8.1. Bullet wound. The cylindrical laceration is much larger in diameter than the .22 calibre bullet which produced it, as a result of the disruptive force of the missile.

tinue in motion momentarily until it impacts against the adjacent bone and dura. Conversely, when the head is sharply accelerated by a blow, the brain lags behind and is thus struck by the moving skull. Since the head pivots on the cervical spine, there is usually an angular or rotational component to the movements, producing differential stresses within the brain substance that tear its substance. The brain is relatively fixed at certain points, notably at the tentorial aperture, so that movements of the hemispheres relative to the brainstem distort and pull upon structures in the midbrain and upper pons. The linear or angular movements of the brain relative to the skull, and of one portion of the brain relative to another, thus account for much of the initial direct cerebral damage. It has been demonstrated, for example, that rapid, forceful flexion or extension of the cervical spine without direct impact to the skull can lead to concussion and cerebral hemorrhage.

There are other factors which may be of importance. Following a blow there is a very sharp rise in intracranial pressure to extremely high levels, lasting for a few milliseconds, that might well produce neuronal damage. Alternating waves of compression and rarefaction may occur in the brain. As the brain moves away from the skull a local transient vacuum occurs, and may be sufficient to lacerate the cortex at that point. These phenomena are extremely short-lived and are difficult to evaluate. In recent years experimental models have been developed in which movements and their distorting effects on the brain are photographed and analyzed through a transparent plastic calvaria following blows of known force; mathematical analysis of the distribution of energy of the impact has been attempted. Following direct impact to the frontal region there is a positive pressure wave in that half of the skull close to the impact while the contrecoup pressure in the occipital area is usually negative. The occurrence of cavitation may prevent a further increase of negative pressure in the contrecoup region. A blow in the occipital region results in opposite pressure effects.

Following injury, some patients show signs pointing to brainstem damage, such as coma, decerebrate rigidity, and disturbances in respiration. Such dysfunction may be the result of brainstem damage or, alternatively, a sequel of raised intracranial pressure with secondary brainstem compression. It is difficult clinically to distinguish between these two situations. Recent studies have shown that there is a group of patients who have relatively mild neurologic deficit at the outset following injury, but later develop a pronounced and progressive rise in intracranial pressure and die within a few days of the injury because of failure of arterial perfusion. Usually the systemic arterial pressure rises in response to an elevation of ventricular fluid pressure, but this is not always so and when it fails, perfusion pressure may fall below a critical level. Methods of controlling elevated intracranial pressure include hyperventilation, osmotic diuretic agents, surgical decompression, and withdrawal of ventricular fluid.

PATHOLOGIC CHANGES IN HEAD INJURY

The effects of head injury may be subdivided as follows:

1. Direct effects of the injury
   a. Skull fractures
   b. Concussion
   c. Contusion and laceration
   d. Hemorrhage
2. Secondary effects
   a. Cerebral swelling
   b. Infection
   c. Intracranial herniations
3. Long-term effects
   a. Focal lesions with permanent neurologic defects
   b. Post-traumatic epilepsy.

Direct Effects of Inury

Fractures of the Skull

Fractures of the bones of the skull are significant in a number of ways:

1. They are a rough indication of the severity and location of the applied force, and hence of possible brain damage.

2. Indriven fragments of bone may lacerate underlying brain or its vessels.

3. Compound fractures and basal fractures involving pharynx and paranasal sinuses may produce cerebrospinal fluid fistulas and also serve as a route of entry for infection.

4. Basal fractures involving foramina containing cranial nerves and major vessels may produce laceration of the contained structures, resulting in paralysis or hemorrhage, respectively.

5. Tearing of meningeal (dural) vessels along a fracture line is the principal cause of extradural hemorrhages.

Concussion

Concussion is defined as temporary loss of consciousness with a variable period of pre- and post-traumatic amnesia, but without permaent detectable clinical damage. Reflex activity of various types—both somatic and autonomic—may be temporarily suppressed or abolished. The patient recovers consciousness within a few seconds or hours, and by definition, has no permanent residual ill effects.

The physiopathology of concussion is inadequately understood. In those few cases adequately studied pathologically when death has occurred from other causes, small lacerations and hemorrhages and focal axonal disruption are frequently encountered in the upper brainstem and hemispheres. Symonds suggested that it is doubtful whether, in concussion, the brain ever escapes some degree of irreversible structural damage. It has proven very difficult to correlate the observed lesions with the severity and duration of the concussive state. It is still unclear whether loss of consciousness is due to a generalized loss of function throughout the cerebral hemispheres or to transient paralysis of a particular region of the brain or brainstem such as the reticular activating formation.

Experimental observations have clearly shown the importance of motion of the brain relative to that of the skull. A blow of very much greater force is required to render an animal comatose if its head is rigidly held than if it is free to move following the blow. The motion imparted to the hemispheres relative to the upper brainstem is considered to disrupt the functioning of the reticular activating system, hence producing unconsciousness. In humans, slow crush injuries, for example a car slipping off a jack onto the head, may not produce immediate unconsciousness even when extensive damage to the brain and skull has occurred.

Contusion and Laceration

Contusion is bruising or pulping of brain tissue as a result of its impact against bone or one of the dural membranes. Laceration, or gross tearing, may be produced by a penetrating object, by indriven bone, by impact against a sharp edge such as the falx cerebri, or by the result of shear forces within the brain itself. In both contusion and laceration, there is discontinuity and death of tissue and disruption of the vascular bed which in turn results in intracerebral and subarachnoid bleeding (Fig. 8.2). Major lacerations of the brainstem or upper cord are immediately fatal.

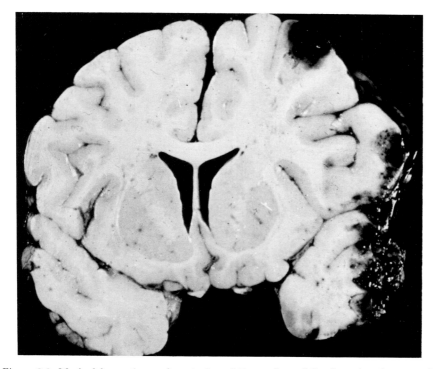

Figure 8.2. Marked laceration and contusion of the surface of the frontal and temporal lobes with hemorrhage and loss of substance. This contrecoup lesion was the result of a blow to the opposite side of the head. The involved hemisphere is also edematous with midline shift.

Contusions are usually at the summit of gyri which impinge against bone—a feature tending to distinguish them from ischemic and anoxic necrosis, which is often most evident in the depths of sulci. The involved area is soft and hemorrhagic (Fig. 8.3), and the dead tissue is gradually removed by the usual process of phagocytosis by macrophages to leave a depressed yellowish (hemosiderin and lipid) fibroglial scar—the "tâche jaune" (Figs. 8.4, 8.5).

The contusions may be at the site of impact—the "coup" lesion—or at the opposite side of the brain—the "contrecoup" lesion. Blows to the occipital area are particularly apt to result in contusion or laceration of the orbital surfaces of the frontal lobes and the temporal poles produced by impact of the moving brain against the irregular bony contours of the anterior fossa and sphenoid ridges. Damage may be minimal at the site of impact, and maximum in the side opposite (Fig. 8.2).

In recent years, a more subtle form of laceration has been recognized. The shear stresses produced by movements of one portion of the brain relative to another may mechanically disrupt the axons, particularly the long fibers traversing the upper brainstem and hemispheres. Gross

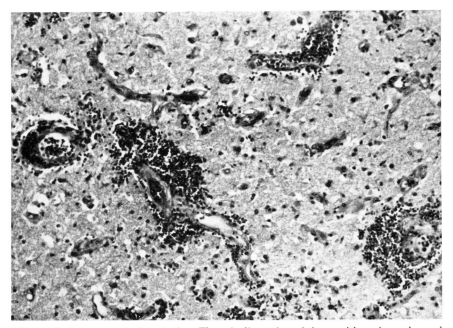

Figure 8.3. Recent cortical contusion. There is disruption of tissue with perivascular and parenchymal hemorrhage, pyknosis of neurons, and early activation of glia. (Hematoxylin-phloxine-saffron, × 125)

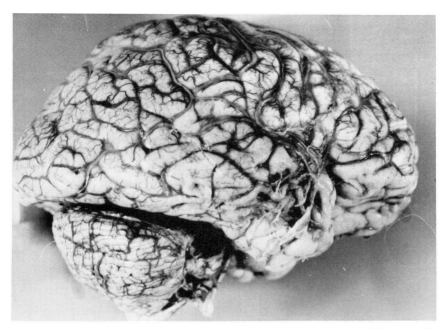

Figure 8.4. Old cortical laceration. On the lateral surface of the temporal lobe is a depressed area with atrophy, loss of cortical substance, and meningeal fibrosis.

examination of the brain often shows no abnormality or only a few small petechiae, the result of concomitant vascular damage; however, microscopic study will show axonal retraction bulbs at the sites where they were severed (Fig. 8.6), and, later, Wallerian degeneration in the involved bundles. These changes, which may be remarkably extensive, are of major importance in the genesis of prolonged coma or other neurologic deficits not due to more massive destructive and easily apparent lesions.

Extradural Hemorrhage

The middle meningeal artery and vein and their branches are embedded in the outer layer of the dura and lie in grooves in the inner aspect of the skull. They are therefore tightly applied to the bones, and are easily torn if a fracture crosses their course. Although the branches of the anterior and posterior meningeal vessels have similar relations, they are less often damaged than are the middle meningeal vessels lying deep to the thin, exposed, easily fractured squamous temporal bone.

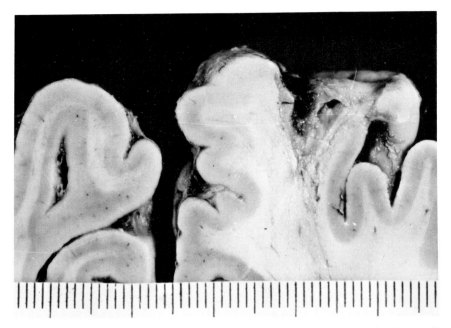

Figure 8.5. Old cortical laceration. The summit of a gyrus has been largely destroyed, leaving a small cavity which extends into the underlying white matter; the fibrotic arachnoid is adherent to the glial wall of the defect. Such fibroglial scars may be epileptogenic.

Hemorrhage from the torn vessels gradually, over minutes or hours, dissects the dura away from the bone, producing a convex lens-shaped hematoma (Fig. 8.7) which compresses the underlying brain, raises the intracranial pressure, and finally produces tentorial herniation with its attendant complications. A volume of about 80 to 100 ml over the vertex, and much less in the posterior fossa, is sufficient to cause death.

The initial head injury may be a major one, but often it is not; the patient regains consciousness, appears well for a short time (the lucid interval), and then gradually develops evidence of elevated intracranial pressure or herniations. An important clinical implication emerges—the physician cannot be too hasty in his decision to release an apparently minor head injury but rather should maintain the patient under careful observation for a period of some hours. Surgical drainage of an epidural hematoma is a relatively simple procedure. The key to successful management is early diagnosis and therapy, before permanent secondary brainstem damage occurs.

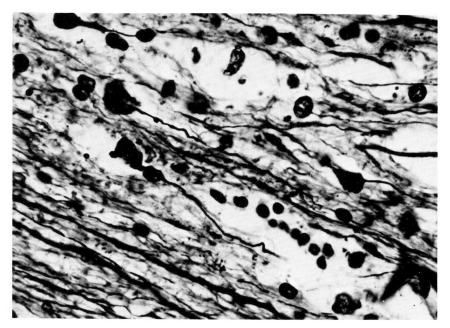

Figure 8.6. Shear injury in centrum semiovale. There is focal disruption of tissue, with axonal tearing and retraction bulb formation. Foci of this type were widely distributed in both hemispheres and the upper brainstem. (Bodian, × 300)

Subdural Hemorrhage

Some subdural hemorrhages are venous in origin, arising from the large veins that cross through the subdural space as they pass from the cerebral hemispheres to the major dural sinuses. The veins are torn by the movement of the brain relative to the skull; those along the superior sagittal sinus are most vulnerable. Since an atrophic brain is free to move a greater distance within the skull than is the normal, elderly individuals and others with cerebral atrophy from any cause are much more susceptible to this form of injury. Particularly in these individuals, the injury may have been so slight as to have been forgotten or ignored.

Other subdural hemorrhages are the result of rupture of a subarachnoid hemorrhage (usually from a cortical laceration) through the arachnoid into the subdural space. Some investigators have suggested that the hemorrhage may initially arise between layers of the dura, but this has not gained general acceptance.

Since the bleeding is usually venous, the hematoma grows slowly over several hours or days. When large, acute effects are clinically indis-

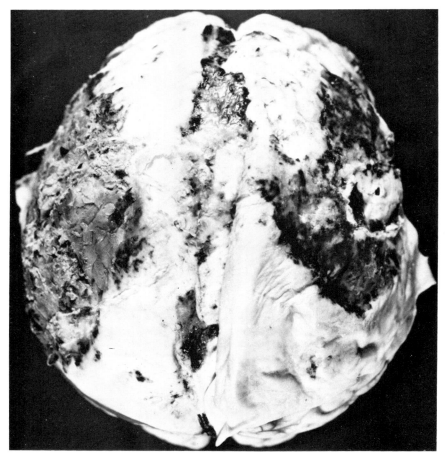

Figure 8.7. Bilateral extradural hematomas. These hematomas were not in themselves sufficiently large to cause a fatal increase in intracranial pressure; death was the result of chest injuries.

tinguishable from those of an epidural hematoma, and the management is similar. However, in contrast to epidural hematomas, subdural bleeding may stop spontaneously before major signs occur. A membrane of granulation tissue grows from the dura at the edges of the hematoma, and over a period of weeks the hematoma becomes encapsulated by a fibrovascular membrane (Fig. 8.8) and the contained blood gradually breaks down. Unfortunately, the osmolarity of the breakdown products is such as to draw in fluid from the small blood vessels in the membrane, and perhaps also cerebrospinal fluid from the adjacent subarachnoid space. In addition, the delicate vessels in the

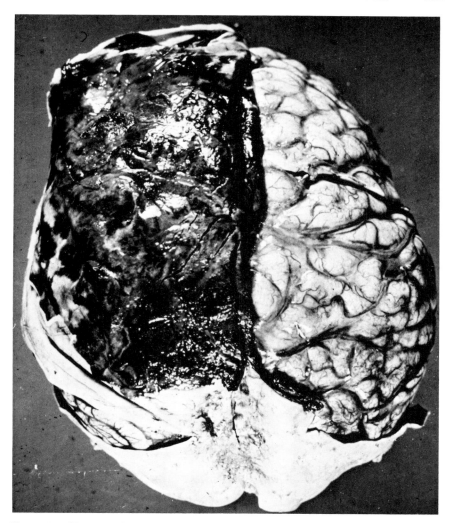

Figure 8.8. Chronic subdural hematoma. The dura covering the right hemisphere has been reflected to the *left* to show its under surface. A large hematoma is covered by a smooth glistening fibrous membrane. Evidence of organization is seen at the lateral edge.

membrane are prone to repeated small additional hemorrhages. As a result, the hematoma slowly expands over several weeks or months, and may reach a volume of 200 to 300 ml before finally producing lethal compression (Fig. 8.9) and herniation. The protracted increase in intracranial mass often fails to produce localizing signs, but instead presents as fluctuating or progressive dementia or behavioral disorders, the

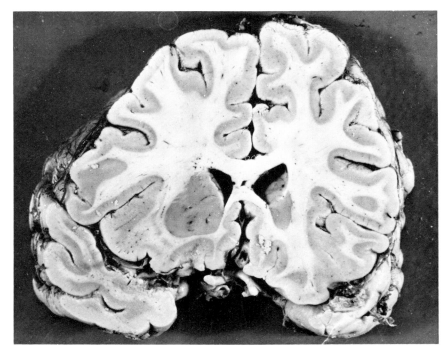

Figure 8.9. Chronic subdural hematoma. An elderly alcoholic female, who had previously undergone portocaval shunting for portal hypertension, suffered a mild head injury 9 months before death. Thereafter, fluctuating levels of awareness were present until her death from liver failure. At autopsy a large (200 ml) subdural hematoma compressed the hemisphere on the *left*. In addition, the discoloration in the putamen on the *left* is due to advanced hepatic encephalopathy, the changes of which were found microscopically in cortex and basal ganglia.

cause of which may easily be overlooked by the unwary clinician. Again, surgical therapy is a relatively simple matter, and the results will be good if treatment is provided before there is compression atrophy of the underlying hemisphere or secondary brainstem damage.

Intracerebral Hematomas

As previously noted, multiple small intracerebral hemorrhages are a common feature of head injury, and are thought to arise from vessels torn by shearing forces within the substance of the brain. Large circumscribed hematomas (Fig. 8.10) are considerably less common, and are probably most often located in the deep white matter of the frontal or temporal lobes following a blow to the occiput. In medicolegal work,

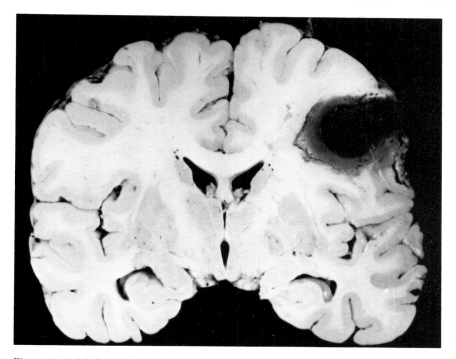

Figure 8.10. Moderate-sized traumatic frontal intracerebral hematoma in association with cortical laceration. There is necrosis with early resorption in the adjacent white matter.

considerable uncertainty occasionally arises as to whether an intracerebral hemorrhage is spontaneous (hypertensive) and the cause of an accident, or is the result of a head injury suffered in the accident.

Because of the disruption of tissue produced by large traumatic intracerebral hematoma and because of its tendency for reaccumulation, it is much less amenable to surgical evacuation than other forms of traumatic intracranial bleeding. Occasionally, drainage is performed in order to attempt to reduce intracranial pressure and preserve brainstem function, but the results are often disappointing.

Indirect Effects of Head Injury

Cerebral Swelling

Following serious injury, swelling of the brain and its attendant effects on intracranial pressure and cerebral blood flow are well recognized major complications.

Cerebral edema occurs in relation to areas of contusion, laceration, and hemorrhage, because of an increase in permeability of vessels adjacent to the lesions. Whether trauma *per se*, in the absence of focal tissue necrosis, produces an alteration in capillary permeability ("traumatic cerebral edema") is not clearly established. However, systemic anoxia or ischemia due to shock, airway obstruction, or respiratory insufficiency have a major role in producing or accentuating cerebral edema in comatose patients and those with multiple injuries, and are in part prevented by careful management on the part of attendants at the scene of an accident.

Vascular congestion as a cause of cerebral swelling and intracranial hypertension has been emphasized in recent years. Autoregulation may be lost following cerebral trauma so that flow varies passively with changes in systemic blood pressure allowing for an increased volume of blood in some circumstances, aggravating the deleterious effects of cerebral edema.

Infection

Bacteria, and rarely, fungi, enter the cranium through compound fractures of the vault or basal fractures which involve the mucosa of the paranasal sinuses, ear, or pharynx. Leakage of cerebrospinal fluid or the finding of air within the skull on x-ray serve to alert the physician to the possibility of infection. Surgical repair of the defect may be necessary.

The infection can involve any of the meningeal spaces or, less often, may take the form of a cerebral abscess. Devitalized tissue probably offers poor resistance to bacterial invasion.

Intracranial Herniations

Although death following head injury occasionally results from primary damage of vital brainstem centers, it is almost always the direct result of increased intracranial pressure with herniations and circulatory stagnation, as discussed in Chapter 3.

Residual Effects of Head Injury

Focal neurologic defects generally improve with time, particularly in children and younger adults in whom the brain seems to have a remarkable capacity to "compensate" functionally for the destroyed tissue. The cranial nerves, unless severed completely, will undergo axonal regeneration and remyelination in a period of several months, although the olfactory and optic nerves, being composed of central nervous tissue, lack this capacity, resulting in troublesome permanent olfactory and visual defects.

In closed head injuries the risk of developing epilepsy is about 5 percent whereas with wounds penetrating the skull and dura, the resulting cortical lesions and associated fibrous and glial scars become epileptogenic foci in an estimated 30 to 50 percent of patients. The risk of chronic post-traumatic epilepsy is much greater in those patients who develop seizures within a few weeks of the injury and in those patients who experience a severe injury as measured by prolonged unconsciousness and post-traumatic amnesia. Surgical excision of the scarred area is sometimes undertaken in the hope that the gliosis occurring in the new defect will be less intense and less epileptogenic than in the more florid traumatic lesions.

Meningeal fibrosis following massive subarachnoid hemorrhage or infection may lead to progressive obstructive hydrocephalus. Unilateral or bilateral enlargement of lateral ventricles may also be the result of cerebral atrophy following destruction of cortical tissue or of axons in white matter. Diabetes insipidus or other symptoms of pituitary or hypothalamic dysfunction are rare chronic complications of head injury.

The majority of head injuries are associated with only minor concussion yet, frequently, even mild injuries are followed by a post-concussion syndrome in which the patient complains of bothersome headache and dizziness, the latter often made worse by changes in position and associated with positional nystagmus. Such symptoms usually arise initially on the basis of mild structural damage such as subpial bleeding and labyrinthine dysfunction, but they may be complicated by the patient's anxiety or the emotional effects of protracted litigation.

INJURIES OF THE SPINAL CORD

Spinal cord injuries may be the direct result of penetrating injuries by bullets, knives, or similar objects. Brown-Sequard's description, in 1868, of the syndrome of spinal cord hemisection was based on his observation of the neurologic defects resulting from stab wounds. In civilian life, however, the common type of spinal cord damage is that resulting from dislocation or fracture-dislocation of the vertebral column. These injuries are usually the result of forceful hyperextension or hyperflexion of the spine, and are most frequent in the mobile lower cervical and lumbar regions. Bone and ligaments are forced against the cord, producing a variable degree of contusion or laceration, or more seriously, transection of the cord with hemorrhage and necrosis in the involved segments (Fig. 8.11). The bony deformity may be such as to compress the vascular supply to the cord, adding an ischemic element to the damage.

The pulped, necrotic tissue is removed by phagocytosis and digestion, and a fibroglial scar is formed at the site of damage; resorption of tissue may leave a cystic cavity. Wallerian degeneration occurs in the appropriate ascending and descending tracts. Although some regenerative activity is demonstrable, the axonal sprouts appear to regress after a short time, and no functional recovery occurs. Attempts have been made, both experimentally and in humans, to encourage regeneration by careful accurate apposition of the cord segments and by pharmacologic reduction of inflammation and scar formation, but thus far these measures have not proven to be of significant value. It is not known whether failure of axonal regeneration depends primarily upon a property of the neurons concerned, is the result of the mechanical barrier imposed by the scar tissue, or is due to the failure of the axons to find a suitable metabolic milieu in the distal segment in which to grow.

The clinical consequences of spinal cord injuries will reflect the segment involved and the degree of damage. Transection above C4 produces respiratory paralysis and rapid death.

Severe damage anywhere along the cord will cause both sensory loss and muscle paralysis below the level of the lesion. Although sensory loss may correspond closely to standard patterns of segmental innervation of the skin, it is not uncommon to encounter considerable anatomic

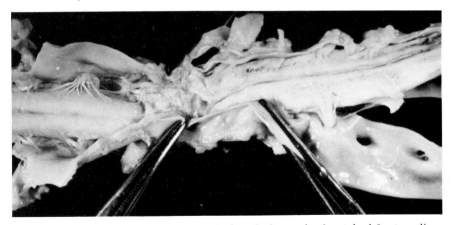

Figure 8.11. Old crush injury of thoracic spinal cord, the result of vertebral fracture-dislocation. A fibroglial scar occupies the site of injury. The patient lived 5 years after the accident, with signs indicating complete spinal cord transection.

variation between patients. More accurate localization is usually determined by defining the uppermost motor segment which is involved. The clinician therefore should be familiar with the major muscles supplied by the segments of the spinal cord. Acute transection of the spinal cord may cause transient spinal shock with loss of all reflexes below the lesion. Reflexes may remain diminished in the affected segment of the cord but, eventually, hyperreflexia and spasticity develop below the level of the lesion. Disturbances in sphincter or sexual function or altered sweating occur as the result of damage to autonomic pathways.

As with major injury elsewhere in the nervous system, little can be done to restore damaged spinal cord tissue, yet careful nursing in special units designed to prevent such complications as decubitus ulcers and bladder infections, along with the incorporation of vigorous physiotherapy programs, can do much to improve the patient's prognosis.

REFERENCES

COURVILLE, C. B. Forensic Neuropathology. Callaghan & Co., Mundelein, Ill., 1964.

COURVILLE, C. B. Trauma to the central nervous system and its membranes. *In* Gradwohl's Legal Medicine. Ed. by F. E. Camps. John Wright & Sons, Ltd., Bristol, 1968.

DENNY-BROWN, D. Brain trauma and concussion. Arch. Neurol. (Chicago) 5:1, 1961.

GOODELL, C. L., AND MEALEY, J., JR. Pathogenesis of chronic subdural hematoma. Experimental studies. Arch. Neurol. (Chicago) 8:429, 1963.

JENNETT, W. B. Epilepsy after Blunt Head Injuries. William Heinemann Medical Books, Ltd., London, 1962.

LANGFITT, T. W., TANNANBAUM, H. M., AND KASSELL, N. F. The etiology of acute brain swelling following experimental head injury. J. Neurosurg. 24:47, 1966.

MORITZ, A. R. The Pathology of Trauma. Lea & Febiger, Philadelphia, 1964.

PEERLESS, S. J., AND REWCASTLE, N. B. Shear injuries of the brain. Canad. Med. Ass. J. 96:577, 1967.

STRITCH, S. Shearing of nerve fibers as a cause of brain damage due to head injury. Lancet 2:443, 1961.

SYMONDS, SIR CHARLES. Concussion and its sequelae. Lancet 1:1, 1962.

WALKER, A. E., CAVENESS, W. F., AND CRITCHLEY, M. The Late Effects of Head Injury. Charles C Thomas, Publisher, Inc., Springfield, Ill., 1969.

9

DEGENERATIVE DISEASES

INTRODUCTION

There is no reasonable scientific basis for bringing together the entities included in this category of disease. The term embraces a group of chronic, slowly progressive diseases of the nervous system of unknown or uncertain etiology, many of them rarely seen, but others, unfortunately, quite common. In recent years, as some of the diseases traditionally placed in this category have been demonstrated to arise from infections, inborn errors of metabolism, etc., the group has been reduced in number, and it may in time disappear. The entities which still remain provide intriguing problems for current investigators able to apply new approaches and methods of study to these problems.

In the classical approach to neuropathology, diseases included as being "degenerative" have certain poorly-defined features in common:

1. The etiology is unknown. Some have important genetic factors; others do not.

2. Many selectively affect certain groups of neurons and/or long tracts with shared or related functional properties—hence the term, "system degenerations."

3. Most are primarily diseases of neurons or their axons or both; changes in myelin sheaths and glia appear to be secondary.

4. They are slowly and relentlessly progressive. Some occur in infancy or childhood and others in later life, but the age of onset and rate of progression are roughly similar among persons with the same entity.

5. Evidence of inflammation is characteristically absent.

There are many clinical syndromes or diseases classified as degenerative, and much disagreement exists regarding the classification of the less common ones, based often on reports of single or a few cases with incomplete documentation. Only a few well-established entities will be considered here; the principles learned are applicable to the analysis of the other syndromes as they are encountered and documented.

A convenient and useful classification is one based on the sites of predominant involvement and principal clinical features, although it must be emphasized that lesions are *not* necessarily confined to these areas.

Examples to be discussed:

1. Degeneration of cerebral cortex: Alzheimer's disease / Pick's disease

2. Degeneration of basal ganglia: Parkinson's disease / Huntington's chorea

3. Degeneration of motor system: Motor neuron disease

4. Degeneration of spino-cerebellar system: Friedreich's ataxia / Olivopontocerebellar degeneration

5. Degeneration of peripheral nerves: Peroneal muscular atrophy

DEGENERATIONS OF CEREBRAL CORTEX

Alzheimer's Disease

This is a very common disease of middle and late life and is the principal cause of the clinical syndromes of pre-senile and senile dementia. Although the term "Alzheimer's disease" (in recognition of the clinical report by Alzheimer in 1907) was first used by Kraepelin in 1910 to indicate those cases with onset in middle age (pre-senile dementia), most would now agree that this separation by age has no basis in pathology and offers few advantages.

The disease begins insidiously and is characterized by a generalized deterioration in mental functions. Loss of memory and carelessness in dress and conduct appear early. The patient lacks foresight, appears disoriented, and may show sudden changes of mood with easy distractibility. Aphasia and dysarthria are common and epileptic seizures may occur. Inability to recognize objects (agnosia) or failure to carry out purposive movements on command in the absence of paralysis (apraxia) may appear. Spastic weakness with hyperreflexia and urinary and fecal incontinence appear in the later stages. The duration of the disease may vary from 1 to 10 or more years, with some patients showing rapid deterioration within 1 year whereas others have a slower decline and may require only minimal care for a number of years.

Etiology

The cause is unknown. Although a few familial cases have been reported, most occur sporadically. Viruses have not been found in ultrastructural or transmission studies. In the older literature, much emphasis was placed on the concept that the disease is one of premature or accelerated "aging" of the brain, based principally on the observations that similar changes are encountered to a mild degree in the brains of about half of elderly but functionally "normal" individuals. Whether these changes are truly the result of aging or represent a minimal subclinical variant of the same disease is debatable; an analogy with clinically inapparent atherosclerosis comes to mind in this regard.

Pathologic Changes

The principal lesions are distributed diffusely and symmetrically throughout the cerebral cortex with minimal involvement of basal ganglia or other subcortical structures. There is a tendency to preferential involvement of the frontal and temporal lobes (Fig. 9.1) with the hippocampi usually severely affected. Gyri appear narrowed, sulci

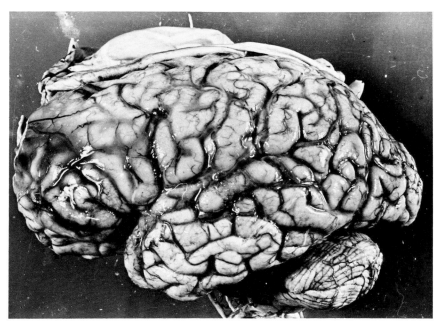

Figure 9.1. Alzheimer's disease. There is moderate atrophy of the frontal and anterior temporal lobes with widening of sulci and mild meningeal fibrosis.

widened, and ventricles dilated (Fig. 9.2), features shared with other atrophic cortical processes and clinically demonstrable by pneumoencephalography (Fig. 9.3). The meninges are often somewhat fibrotic.

Histologically, there is widespread loss of neurons, notably from the third and fifth cortical layers (Fig. 9.4), and proliferation of fibrous astrocytes—findings present in several of the "degenerative" diseases of the central nervous system. The dementia is undoubtedly a reflection of the degree of neuronal loss and dysfunction. In addition, however, two changes are found which characterize the pathology of Alzheimer's disease despite the fact that neither is specific to it:

Neurofibrillary Degeneration of Neurons. The cell bodies of neurons are distended and their nuclei are displaced by the accumulation within the cytoplasm of skeins and loops of argyrophilic fibers (Fig. 9.5) which by electron microscopy are composed of dense arrays of parallel "twisted tubules" about 220 Å in diameter. The origin of the twisted tubules is unknown; they are morphologically distinct from both micro-

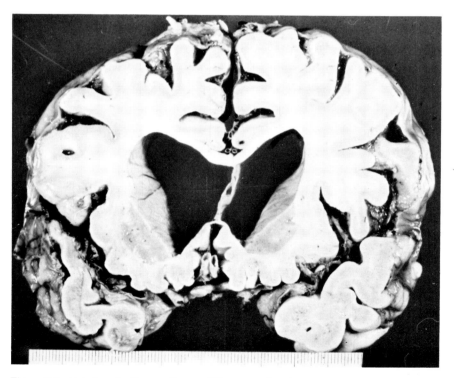

Figure 9.2. Alzheimer's disease. Severe diffuse atrophy of cortex and white matter, and marked ventricular dilatation. Gyri are narrowed and sulci gape widely.

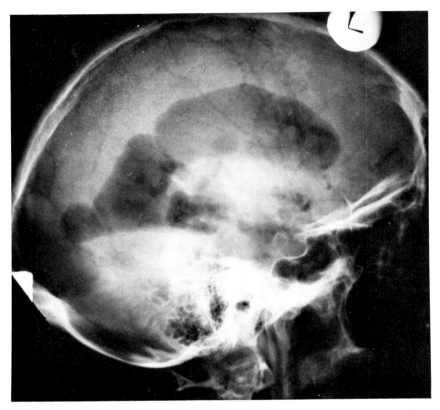

Figure 9.3. Alzheimer's disease. Female, age 65. Increasing dementia for 2 years. Pneumoencephalogram shows diffuse severe ventricular enlargement, particularly of the body and anterior horn of the lateral ventricle.

tubules and neurofilaments and also from the neurofibrillary tangles of 100 Å filaments produced experimentally in neurons by spindle inhibitors and alumina. Aggregates of 220 Å twisted tubules are also present in neurons in some cases of post-encephalitic Parkinsonism and Pick's disease. It has been suggested that the twisted tubules may arise from re-assembly of breakdown products of normal microtubules.

Amyloid ("Senile") Plaques. Plaques are small extracellular deposits of amyloid, surrounded by a few macrophages and by rather swollen, varicose neurites containing numerous secondary lysosomes (Figs. 9.4, 9.5). Terry and co-workers believe that first there is focal degeneration of neurites (notably dendrites) followed by a phagocytic response; the macrophages appear to form the amyloid protein locally. At the ultrastructural level, the deposits contain 100 Å filaments indistinguish-

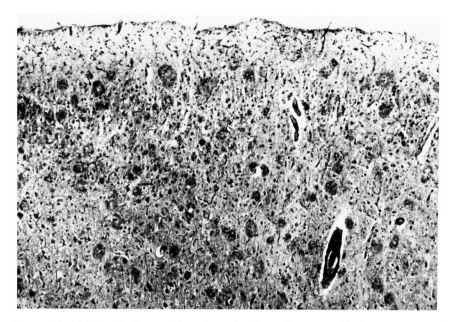

Figure 9.4. Alzheimer's disease. There is marked loss of neurons with the appearance of cortical disorganization. The numerous small nuclei in the outer layers are largely those of astrocytes. A large number of spherical dense senile plaques are scattered throughout all layers. (Bielschowsky, × 45)

able from naturally occurring or experimentally induced systemic amyloid.

Amyloid plaques are found in almost all elderly individuals but are very numerous only when clinical dementia and detectable neuronal fallout are present. However, they are also usually present in small numbers in persons of apparently normal intellect. It has been suggested that plaques are a relatively non-specific reaction to individual or focal cortical neuronal degeneration from several causes. The occasional concentration of amyloid plaques near old infarcts may support this hypothesis. However, in numerous other diseases with neuronal loss, plaques are not a feature.

Many cases with prominent amyloid plaques also have amyloid deposits in small cerebral blood vessels (congophilic angiopathy), and there is a statistical association with perivascular amyloid deposits in myocardium. However, there is no apparent relationship of plaques with the usual primary, secondary, and familial forms of systemic amyloidosis. In these latter conditions, deposits may be found in meninges, choroid plexus, cerebral blood vessels, and peripheral nerves.

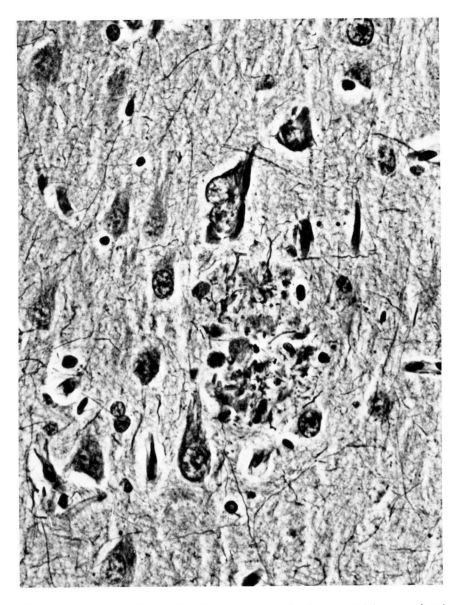

Figure 9.5. Alzheimer's disease. Near the *center* is a senile plaque containing several varicose neuronal processes and clumps of homogeneous material representing amyloid. The
neurons immediately above the plaque contain bundles of dense argyrophilic fibers (neurofibrillary degeneration) which have displaced the nuclei to the left. (Bodian, × 400)

Alzheimer's disease is an extremely common cause for dementia in middle-aged and elderly patients. Although the cause is unknown, the evidence available would suggest that the pathologic changes should not be considered as part of normal aging but, rather, a manifestation of a relatively common disease which may often remain limited in severity and produce no significant clinical findings.

Pick's Disease

Pick's disease is an uncommon cause of dementia. The clinical pattern of progressive dementia, memory loss, and occasional focal signs is similar to the other late-onset cortical degenerations, although some symptoms, such as loss of normal social inhibition and marked mood swings, may suggest early and more severe impairment of frontal lobe function.

Two epidemiologic features are worthy of note. First, the disease is at least twice as common in women as in men. Secondly, although most cases occur sporadically, the familial incidence in some series is quite striking with involvement in as many as five generations. The etiology is, however, unknown, and no metabolic disturbances have been identified.

The pathologic findings are quite distinctive. The brain exhibits cortical atrophy which may be diffuse but is often very severe in one or both frontal and temporal lobes with sparing of the paracentral areas (Fig. 9.6). Very severe atrophy of the anterior one-third of the superior temporal gyrus with sparing of the posterior portions is commonly noted. Some degree of atrophy, occasionally severe, is present in basal ganglia as well.

There is moderate to severe loss of neurons in the affected areas and gliosis is usually intense (Fig. 9.7). Some of the surviving neurons are greatly distended by distinctive large cytoplasmic inclusions which displace the nuclei to the periphery (Fig. 9.8). Their nature and significance are unknown; they are composed of random, closely packed filaments of tubules 70 to 100 Å in diameter without a limiting membrane, and are composed in part of protein. Whether this accumulation is due to an intrinsic metabolic defect or to the action of an exogenous agent is unknown.

DEGENERATIONS OF BASAL GANGLIA

Although certain signs and symptoms are diagnostic of disease of the extrapyramidal system, our knowledge of extrapyramidal function in

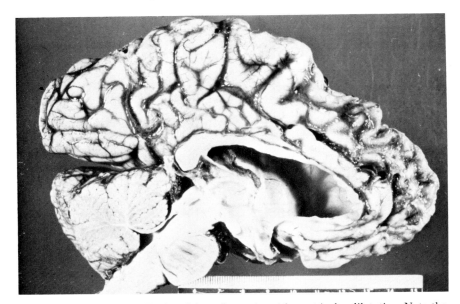

Figure 9.6. Pick's disease. Profound frontal atrophy with ventricular dilatation. Note the sharp demarcation between affected and non-affected frontal cortex.

the normal person is limited, and any advance in our understanding will require much additional correlation of anatomic, physiologic, and neurochemical factors. Not only are anatomic and other facets ill-understood at this time, but the symptoms characteristic of human disease are often unique to biped man and cannot easily be duplicated in studies of experimental animals.

The extrapyramidal system consists of a number of interconnected nuclear masses located deep in the cerebral hemispheres and in the brainstem. These nuclei are the caudate, putamen, globus pallidus, red nucleus, subthalamic nucleus, and substantia nigra. The caudate and putamen receive input from the cerebral cortex, thalamus, and midbrain. The globus pallidus provides the main efferent pathway of the basal ganglia, sending fibers to thalamus, substantia nigra, red nucleus, and subthalamic nucleus. Through this network there is integration of labyrinthine, body righting, visual, and other sensory input with the motor system. The extrapyramidal system is necessary for the maintenance of normal posture and locomotion which it modulates through its connections with cerebral cortex, thalamus, cerebellum, and labyrinthine nuclei.

Diseases involving the basal ganglia are often rather diffuse in their location and it is difficult to correlate clinical signs with damage to

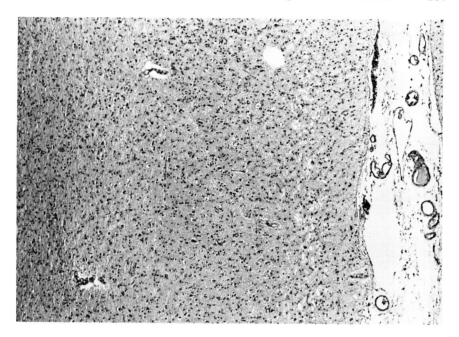

Figure 9.7. Pick's disease. Severe neuronal loss and gliosis, particularly in the outer half of the cortex. The spongy or reticulated appearance of the outer cortex is a reflection of the severity of the damage. (Hematoxylin-phloxine-saffron, × 45)

specific anatomic sites. There is a broad range of symptoms but their essential components consist of alterations in posture and the occurrence of involuntary movements. Although numerous types of involuntary movements may be seen, they are interrelated, and one patient may demonstrate a number of movement and postural disturbances during the course of a chronic disease. Involuntary movements may appear as part of an acute reversible disease, such as Sydenham's chorea, or complicate longstanding and static brain damage, such as the athetosis of infantile hemiplegia, or be part of a slowly progressive degenerative disease, such as those discussed below. Common signs in extrapyramidal disease include athetosis, chorea, dystonia, tremor, rigidity, and hypokinesia.

Athetosis refers to an instability of posture characterized by continual writhing movements, seen best in the upper extremity and consisting of a slow alteration between extension and flexion of fingers, often with trapping of the thumb under the index finger. Lips, tongue, and jaw are also often involved, with intermittent flexion of the neck. Chorea consists of a sudden lapse of posture and accentuation of as-

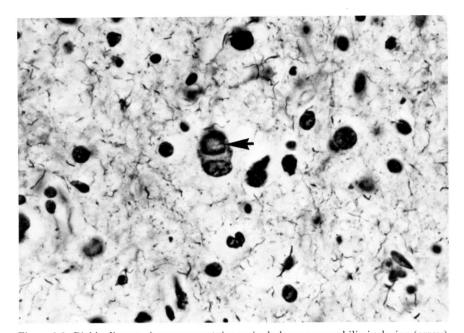

Figure 9.8. Pick's disease. A neuron contains a single large argyrophilic inclusion (*arrow*) characteristic of the disease. (Bodian, × 450)

sociated body movements. The sudden unpredictable movements may occur at rest or during active use of an extremity. Hypotonia (diminished resistance to passive movement) is frequently associated with chorea. Dystonia is the persistent maintenance of an abnormal posture often associated with increased resting muscle tone (hypertonia). It may take various forms, such as the flexion dystonia of Parkinson's disease, or hemiplegic dystonia.

Tremor is a rhythmic alteration of contraction in opposing muscle groups and in extrapyramidal disease is characteristically present at rest. It often begins in the thumb and adjacent fingers and disappears with movement, only to return shortly after the limb maintains a new posture. Although such a tremor may be greatly modified by removing the sensory input from a limb, such an experiment only serves to demonstrate the continual interplay of sensory and motor elements in determining movement. In some instances, tremor may represent the release of an intrinsic thalamic rhythm.

Rigidity is another aspect of altered motor function commonly seen with extrapyramidal disease. It is manifest by increased resistance to passive movement which is relatively constant throughout the range of movement, and will have a cogwheel character when an underlying tremor is superimposed.

Denny-Brown interprets the involuntary movements of extrapyramidal diseases in terms of released proprioceptive reactions, and has shown the way that the abnormal postures and movements can be modified by changing body contact with surfaces or altering body position in space. The movements of athetosis he considers as aspects of released grasping and avoiding reactions.

Disease in the basal ganglia may influence function at lower levels in the motor system in terms of the large alpha motor fibers innervating skeletal muscle and the smaller gamma fibers innervating intrafusal (spindle) muscle fibers. Difficulty in initiating a movement (hypokinesia) is a disturbing symptom for many patients and often presents as difficulty in getting up from a chair, walking, or using an extremity independently. This difficulty in movement may be due to a defect in a gamma starter mechanism which precedes alpha motor activity in normal movements. Ward has suggested that as a result of extrapyramidal disease there may be a depression of gamma activity and enhancement of alpha firing. He suggests that disease of the extrapyramidal system may interrupt the excitatory neurons to the gamma circuit leaving the inhibitory ones intact, producing relative depression of gamma and enhancement of alpha activity. This inhibitory bias might account for hypokinesia; defective negative feedback in a gamma loop system could lead to oscillation and tremor.

Parkinson's Disease

The syndrome of tremor at rest, bradykinesia, and extrapyramidal rigidity appearing in middle-aged or elderly individuals constitutes Parkinson's syndrome (Fig. 9.9). The usual idiopathic form is called Parkinson's disease or paralysis agitans. Many instances of Parkinson's syndrome developed in persons who suffered encephalitis lethargica during the 1917–1920 pandemic (post-encephalitic Parkinsonism), but these are now less frequently seen. As will be discussed subsequently, certain drugs may produce a Parkinson-like syndrome which usually clears when they are withdrawn.

The essential pathologic change in the idiopathic and post-encephalitic forms is the loss of neurons from certain of the pigmented (melanin-containing) neurons of the brainstem, notably the substantia nigra and locus ceruleus (Fig. 9.10). Inconstant changes found in the globus pallidus and putamen are generally considered to be secondary or the result of coincidental vascular disease. There is no good evidence of

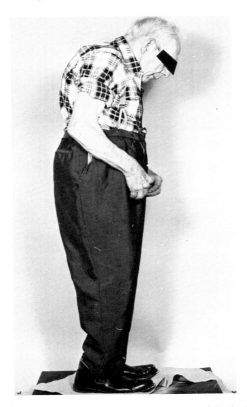

Figure 9.9. Parkinson's disease. Note the characteristic immobile facies and the posture of flexion of neck and all extremities. Patient had great difficulty initiating walking (brady-kinesia). Rigidity lessened somewhat following treatment with L-DOPA.

cortical degeneration in this disease. Surviving neurons in the sub-stantia nigra and other nuclei often contain large spherical, laminated cytoplasmic inclusions (Lewy bodies), the significance of which is un-known (Fig. 9.11). Neurofibrillary tangles are occasionally present in the idiopathic disease, but are more common in the post-encephalitic syndrome in which Lewy bodies are unusual.

Neurons of the substantia nigra are believed to release the catechola-mine dopamine as a transmitter substance. Their axons are thought to terminate predominantly in the basal ganglia, particularly in the caudate nucleus and putamen where they exert an inhibitory action. In Parkinson's disease, there is marked reduction in dopamine in these areas, corresponding to loss of the dopamine-producing neurons in the substantia nigra. Since the highest concentration of the transmitter is

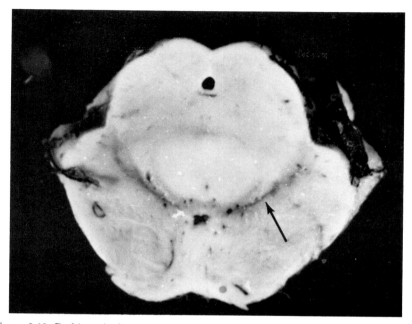

Figure 9.10. Parkinson's disease. Section of lower midbrain showing shrinkage and loss of pigment from the substantia nigra (*arrow*), reflecting neuronal loss and gliosis in this nucleus.

in the terminal axons, the reduction is most evident in the caudate nucleus and putamen. In an attempt to replenish cerebral dopamine stores, its precursor, L-DOPA (dihydroxyphenylalanine), has been given to patients with Parkinsonism. Dopamine does not easily penetrate the blood-brain barrier, but L-DOPA appears to pass through the capillary endothelium by a specific carrier mechanism. If adequate decarboxylase activity is present in the striatum, dopamine will be formed from administered L-DOPA. It is not known whether dopamine or one of its metabolites contains the active anti-Parkinsonian agent, but a large percentage of Parkinsonian patients experience improvement in rigidity, akineasia, and, to a lesser degree, tremor following treatment with L-DOPA.

A number of drugs may induce a Parkinsonian syndrome when given in sufficiently large amounts. Reserpine depletes the endogenous central nervous system stores of 5-hydroxytryptamine and dopamine and causes release of norepinephrine and other cerebral amines. If reserpine is given in large doses, it may induce not only a fairly common depressive reaction or other psychic disturbances, but a Parkinsonian syndrome as well. Chlorpromazine and haloperidol also produce Parkinsonian syndromes, possibly through a blockade of catecholamine receptors, which again could lead to the removal of normal inhibitory effects upon the extrapyramidal system. Such drug-induced syndromes are slightly more common in females and in patients within the age range of idiopathic paralysis agitans. Such an iatrogenic Parkinsonian syndrome is occasionally irreversible in spite of removal of the offending drug.

There is evidence that acetylcholine is an excitatory transmitter in the striatum. Under normal conditions some of the inherent activity of the striatum may be inhibited by the pathways which are damaged in diseases of the extrapyramidal system. Release of such inhibition may then be manifest clinically in the form of the symptoms described above. This mechanism could explain the improvement which has long been observed to occur in patients given belladonna and other anticholinesterase agents and would be in keeping with the antagonistic effect of atropine to acetylcholine. Trihexyphenidyl blocks acetylcholine at certain cerebral synaptic sites and remains a useful anti-Parkinsonian

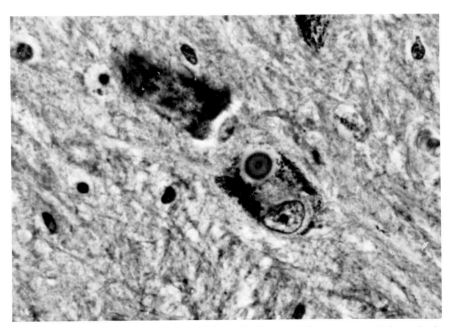

Figure 9.11. Parkinson's disease. A surviving melanin-containing neuron contains a single spherical laminated cytoplasmic inclusion (Lewy body). (Luxol fast blue-hematoxylin-eosin (LFB-HE), × 450)

drug. Conversely, cholinergic drugs have been shown to aggravate Parkinsonian symptoms.

It has been recognized for many years that if a patient with Parkinsonism suffers a stroke, he experiences improvement in tremor and rigidity on the involved side of the body. It was thought that this improvement was due to interruption of the corticospinal tracts, but in recent years, improvement has been seen to follow such varied lesions as undercutting of the cerebral cortex, destruction of the deep cerebellar nuclei, or damage to the globus pallidus or thalamus. The development of stereotactic surgery has enabled neurosurgeons to produce accurately localized lesions within the brain and favored targets in Parkinsonism have been globus pallidus and the ventral lateral nucleus of thalamus. Both of these structures are important efferent pathways for the extrapyramidal system, and lesions in these regions presumably upset an abnormal motor balance developed during the evolution of the disease. The beneficial effects of such lesions, however, are often transient and tremor may return after a few months.

Huntington's Chorea

Huntington's chorea usually presents in a characteristic clinical fashion. It is usually inherited as a Mendelian dominant. Sporadic cases occasionally occur, due possibly to genetic mutations although some may represent distinct and unrelated diseases. They all have similar clinical and pathologic features.

Symptoms and signs do not usually appear until the fourth or fifth decade, by which time the individual has had the opportunity to pass the genetic defect to the next generation. Occasionally, the onset is in childhood or adolescence or delayed until old age. The disease usually begins with the appearance of quick choreic movements which the patient may attempt to conceal. Writhing athetoid movements then appear, often including a characteristic sideways movement of the head. Occasionally, in the later stages, increasing rigidity may appear with the development of dystonic postures. Dementia, characterized by disturbances in mood and judgment and alterations in behavior, usually develops in association with the movement disorder. In some families, the dementia component appears early and is severe; in others, involuntary movements may be present for years without severe impairment of intellect. As the disease evolves, however, the majority of cases show both the typical involuntary movements and gradually increasing dementia.

Examination of the brain reveals moderate to severe frontal and parietal atrophy on the basis of cortical neuronal loss and gliosis. On section, there is ventricular enlargement and severe atrophy of the caudate nucleus and putamen, with milder changes in the subthalamic nucleus and other basal ganglia and brainstem nuclei (Fig. 9.12). Shrinkage of the head of the caudate may flatten or make concave the normally convex outline of the lateral wall of the anterior horn of the ventricles, a feature occasionally evident by pneumoencephalography. There are no specific cellular inclusions. No specific biochemical abnormalities are known.

DEGENERATION OF THE MOTOR SYSTEM
Motor Neuron Disease

Motor neuron disease is one of the commoner system degenerations. The majority of cases occur sporadically, although about 5 to 10 percent of North American instances are familial on the basis of dominant inheritance. There are no known biochemical changes. No infective agents have been isolated.

The disease presents most frequently in the fifth decade of life. It has

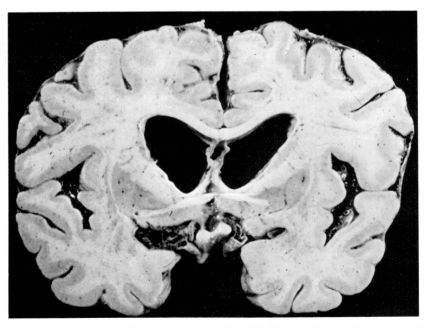

Figure 9.12. Huntington's chorea. Severe atrophy of the head of the caudate nucleus bilaterally, with ventricular enlargement. Mild cortical atrophy is also evident.

an insidious onset and early symptoms will correspond to the region in the central nervous system first affected. The principal changes are those of shrinkage, chromatolysis, and, finally, loss of anterior horn cells, particularly in the cervical and lumbar spinal segments, and of the motor nuclei of the lower cranial nerves (Fig. 9.13). As well, the corticospinal tracts and their cells of origin in the pre-central gyri degenerate and disappear. The clinical picture is thus one of weakness with a mixture of signs of upper motor neuron dysfunction (spasticity, hyperreflexia, Babinski's sign) and lower motor neuron signs (absent reflexes and wasting). A common mode of presentation is for weakness and muscle wasting to appear in the small muscles of one hand spreading to the same shoulder, and then, frequently, to the tongue and bulbar muscles. Eventually, the disease becomes generalized, with severe paralysis of limbs and disturbances of speech and swallowing.

Widespread fasciculations (brief twitches of single motor units) are common and are easily seen in the tongue and superficial skeletal muscles. The appearance of fasciculations in motor neuron disease is

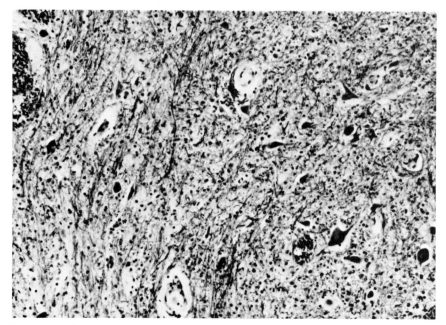

Figure 9.13. Motor neuron disease. The field encompasses the width of a thoracic anterior horn in which there is loss of neurons, marked shrinkage of those remaining, and intense glial proliferation. (LFB-HE, × 125)

thought to be a reflection of active disease in the anterior horn cell or the proximal portion of its axon. Fasciculations may also be induced in normal persons by anti-cholinesterase drugs and at other times appear spontaneously in the absence of disease (benign fasciculation). The mechanism producing fasciculations remains unclear and a distinction between the benign and pathologic forms is best made by considering the examination of the patient as a whole.

Fibrillation potentials (rapid contractions of single muscle fibers) may be detected on the electromyogram and are an additional indication of denervation. Fibrillation potentials appear 10 days to 2 weeks following removal of the nerve supply to a muscle, and will appear in other settings of denervation. An exception is the fibrillation potentials which may be recorded during an attack of hyperkalemic periodic paralysis where, presumably, alterations in electrolytes are important.

Although motor involvement dominates the pathologic picture, less severe degenerative changes are rather widespread throughout the lateral and anterior columns of the spinal cord. This is particularly true of the uncommon familial cases in which Clarke's column and the spinocerebellar tracts are frequently conspicuously involved, suggesting a link with the familial spinocerebellar degenerations. Posterior columns are usually spared, although they have been involved in some familial cases. Patients frequently complain of muscle cramps, especially in the early stages of the disease, but sensory signs and symptoms are generally conspicuous by their absence. A diagnosis of motor neuron disease is essentially untenable in the presence of persistent sensory changes.

The disease is relentlessly progressive, death occurring within 3 to 5 years, usually the result of paralysis of bulbar muscles. When the bulbar and facial muscles are involved early ("progressive bulbar palsy"), life expectancy is much shorter. The prognosis is best in those patients in whom the disease appears confined to the lower motor neurons for a long period of time.

The distribution of nerve cell loss somewhat resembles that in poliomyelitis. A few cases of a motor neuron disease-like syndrome have been described in persons who had poliomyelitis years previously, raising the possibility of persistence of the virus and its subsequent re-activation to produce slowly progressive destruction.

Infantile spinal muscular atrophy (Werdnig-Hoffmann disease) is an uncommon familial disease in which there is progressive loss of cells from anterior horns and the motor cranial nuclei, beginning in infancy or childhood. In contrast to motor neuron disease, changes in spinal tracts are minimal.

SPINOCEREBELLAR DEGENERATIONS

Progressive degenerations affecting ascending and descending tracts in the brainstem and spinal cord, and the cerebellum and its connections, occur both sporadically and as inherited disorders. Numerous syndromes are described both clinically and pathologically; some become manifest in childhood or adolescence, and others occur in adults or the elderly. In a few types, there is also widespread involvement of other areas of the central nervous system, including retina, cortex, and basal ganglia. Clinically, these patients demonstrate various combinations of progressive spinal or cerebellar ataxia, spastic quadriparesis, sensory loss, and, occasionally, blindness, dementia, and extrapyramidal signs. In the inherited forms, the members of a given family tend to show quite similar features which differ somewhat in detail from the pattern seen in other unrelated families. As a result, the presently used rather complex classifications are less than adequate and will not be outlined in this book. Readers interested in further details are referred to the standard neurology texts.

One example which usually presents in a characteristic clinical way is Friedreich's ataxia. In some families, it is inherited as a dominant trait, but in others it is recessive. The onset is usually in childhood, and survival beyond early adult life is uncommon. Cerebellar ataxia of the legs is followed by involvement of the upper extremities and dysarthria. Gait is further compromised by weakness and by impairment of vibration and position sense, and the majority of patients soon become confined to chair or bed. Some patients show optic atrophy and deafness has been described. Pathologically, there is severe loss of axons and gliosis of posterior columns, corticospinal tracts, and spinocerebellar tracts, and minimal cortical atrophy of the cerebellum. Some patients also exhibit a progressive myocardiopathy leading to cardiac enlargement and failure; diabetes occurs with greater incidence than in the general population. These latter features suggest a widespread effect of the genetic error within each patient.

Another apparent entity is olivopontocerebellar degeneration of Déjerine and Thomas. It occurs in either middle or late adult life in either a sporadic or familial fashion with the former predominating. Although examination will reveal a mixture of more or less symmetrical cerebellar and pyramidal signs, the clinical features are not specific and a diagnosis rests on the pathologic demonstration of severe neuronal loss in the pontine nuclei and the olives. The cerebellar cortex has a mild loss of Purkinje cells, but there is marked pallor of myelin staining in the middle cerebellar peduncles and cerebellar white matter. There is often degeneration of basal ganglia leading to extrapyramidal signs; as well, cortical neuronal loss may be responsible for dementia.

DEGENERATION OF PERIPHERAL NERVES

Peroneal Muscular Atrophy

There are several familial polyneuropathies described, and many of these suffer the same uncertainties of classification as do the spinocerebellar degenerations, with which some appear to overlap. Acceptable classifications will result from clear definition of the biochemical defect involved.

Peroneal muscular atrophy (Marie-Charcot-Tooth disease) serves as an example of this group and illustrates some of the problems involved. It is a very slowly progressive chronic degeneration of peripheral nerves, usually occurring on the basis of dominant inheritance. Most patients present in childhood or adolescence with a motor neuropathy involving the feet and lower legs, with moderate to marked wasting of muscles of the lower legs, acquired equinus or varus deformities of the foot, and foot drop. There may be lesser involvement of both superficial and deep sensation. Often the changes are not incapacitating, or are readily compensated by simple orthopedic devices. In others, however, there is progressive disabling paralysis and wasting which also involves the hands and arms. Rarely, there may be evidence of spinal cord lateral and posterior column involvement to produce syndromes reminiscent of Friedreich's ataxia.

The pathologic changes in peripheral nerves consist of loss of axons and myelin sheaths, endoneurial fibrosis, and proliferation of Schwann cells. The latter cells often form overlapping cylindrical whorls which in cross section have the appearance of onion-bulbs. The proliferative changes may be of sufficient degree that subcutaneous nerves become palpable as firm cords. Skeletal muscles show the changes of chronic denervation. Older reports of primary myopathic changes appear to have been based on lack of awareness of the severity and range of changes produced by longstanding partial denervation. Spinal cord changes are quite variable. There may be reduction in anterior horn cells, and posterior columns; corticospinal and spinocerebellar tracts may exhibit mild degenerative changes.

CONCLUSIONS

The system degenerations, particularly those with a hereditary basis, present to the clinician a wide spectrum of signs and symptoms and to the pathologist a bewildering array of degenerations of tracts and nuclei. The causes, whether they be biochemical defects or environmental agents, remain undiscovered, and classifications based on descriptions of the clinical or pathologic changes have been unsatisfactory. In general, there are no specific diagnostic tests for this group of diseases, although there may be helpful findings in radiologic, electrophysiologic, and other investigations. It should be apparent, however, that a most careful family history is a key component in the investigation of any slowly progressive neurologic disease.

REFERENCES

DENNY-BROWN, D. The Cerebral Control of Movement. Charles C Thomas, Publisher, Inc., Springfield, Ill., 1966.

DYCK, P. J., AND LAMBERT, E. H. Lower motor and primary sensory neuron diseases with peroneal muscular atrophy. Arch. Neurol. (Chicago) 18:603, 1968.

HIRANO, A., KURLAND, L. T., AND SAYRE, G. P. Familial amyotrophic lateral sclerosis. Arch. Neurol. (Chicago) 16:232, 1967.

HORNYKIEWICZ, O. Dopamine (3-hydroxytyramine) and brain function. Pharmacol. Rev. 18:925, 1966.

McCAUGHEY, W. T. E. The pathologic spectrum of Huntington's chorea. J. Nerv. Ment. Dis. 133:91, 1961.

McDOWELL, F. H., LEE, J. E., SWIFT, T., SWEET, R. D., OGSBURY, J. S., AND KESSLER, J. T. Treatment of Parkinson's syndrome with l-dihydroxyphenylalanine (levodopa). Ann. Intern. Med. 72:29, 1970.

REWCASTLE, N. B., AND BALL, M. J. Electron microscopic structure of the "inclusion bodies" in Pick's disease. Neurology (Minneap.) 18:1205, 1968.

TERRY, R. D. Neuronal fibrous protein in human pathology. J. Neuropath. Exp. Neurol. 30:8, 1971.

TERRY, R. D., GONATAS, N. K., AND WEISS, M. Ultrastructural studies in Alzheimer's presenile dementia. Amer. J. Path. 44:269, 1964.

WEINER, L. P., KONIGSMARK, B. W., STOLL, J., JR., AND MAGLADERY, J. W. Hereditary olivopontocerebellar atrophy with retinal degeneration. Arch. Neurol. (Chicago) 16:364, 1967.

WOLSTENHOLME, G. E. W., AND O'CONNOR, M. (Eds). Alzheimer's Disease and related conditions. J. & A. Churchill, Ltd., London, 1970.

10

INTRACRANIAL NEOPLASMS

Primary intracranial and intraspinal tumors may develop from any of the neuroectodermal cells of the central nervous system or from the associated mesenchymal tissues. Embryonic intracranial inclusions of non-neural tissues also occasionally give rise to tumors.

Neoplasms of the nervous system account for 5 to 10 percent of all tumors and for about 1 to 2 percent of all deaths. They share with the lymphomas and leukemias a tendency to occur with relatively high frequency in children and young adults. In the elderly, metastases to the central nervous system are considerably more frequent than primary tumors.

CLASSIFICATION

None of the numerous classifications of brain tumors has gained universal acceptance, and the complex terminology favored by some workers seems to have served little purpose in relation to our understanding of either the clinical behavior or basic biologic properties of these neoplasms.

The greatly simplified classification presented here serves to illustrate the general pattern of nomenclature, and provides as well a rough impression of incidence expressed as percentages of intracranial neoplasms.

1. Tumors of central neural tissues (45%)
   a. Gliomas
   b. Nerve cell tumors (very rare)
2. Tumors of meninges (15%)
   a. Meningioma
   b. Meningeal sarcoma (rare)
3. Tumors of nerves (5-10%)
   a. Schwannoma
   b. Others (rare)
4. Tumors of pituitary gland (10%)
   a. Adenomas
   b. Carcinoma (very rare)
5. Tumors of blood vessels (3%)
   a. Hemangioblastoma

6. Tumors of embryonic remnants (4%)
   a. Cranipharyngioma
   b. Epidermal cyst
   c. Chordoma
   d. Teratoma
7. Metastatic tumors (10–20%)

GLIOMAS

Gliomas form the largest group of intracranial tumors. Unfortunately, they are rarely curable except in certain specific instances (*vide infra*).

The nomenclature of gliomas is based in part on a resemblance of the tumor cells to the various types of normal glia; hence, there are astrocytomas (the great majority), oligodendrogliomas, ependymomas, and mixed gliomas containing two or more identifiable glial types.

The gliomas are all malignant in that they infiltrate widely and destroy adjacent brain tissue. Demarcation between the tumor and uninvolved tissue is usually indistinct (Fig. 10.1) and surgical removal is thus impossible except in those rare instances when the tumor is so located that a wide margin of apparently normal tissue surrounding the tumor can be removed. The astrocytomas particularly tend to invade the corpus callosum to spread to the other hemisphere, and infiltrate along axonal bundles for considerable distances.

Any of the gliomas may invade the meninges and ventricular surfaces and become disseminated through the cerebrospinal fluid pathways. However, in the absence of surgery, remote metastases to other organs or lymph nodes are almost unknown. Following craniotomy, malignant cells may invade the scalp and very occasionally spread through the systemic circulation. As a general rule, a tumor with visceral metastases is almost certainly *not* a glioma.

Gliomas exhibit widely varying growth rates, and there is fairly good correlation between the prognosis and the histologic appearance in individual cases when allowance is made as well for other factors such as location within the nervous system, the patient's age, and the severity of secondary changes such as edema and hemorrhage. A commonly used, conceptually simple method of expressing the histologic appearance is that of grading. Grade I astrocytomas are very slow-growing tumors, the cells of which closely resemble normal or hypertrophied astrocytes (Fig. 10.2), and which have a mean survival period of 8 years from the first symptoms. At the other extreme, Grade IV astrocytomas are among the most rapidly fatal tumors to occur in man. The cells show gross pleomorphism, with marked nuclear hyperchromasia, numerous tumor giant cells, and many mitoses (Fig. 10.3). Necrosis and

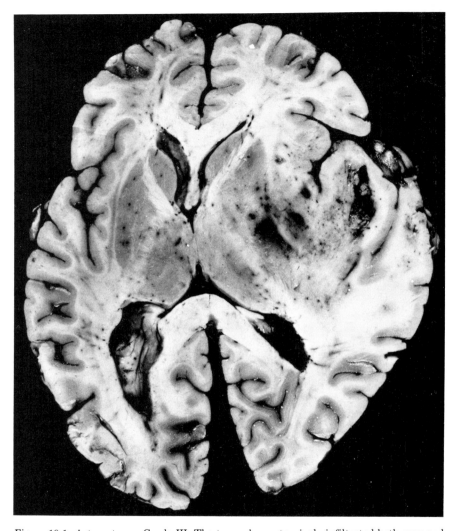

Figure 10.1. Astrocytoma, Grade III. The tumor has extensively infiltrated both gray and white matter of the temporal and parietal lobes and the putamen, globus pallidus, thalamus, and internal capsule. Extensive necrosis and hemorrhage are commonly seen in the more malignant gliomas. The tumor margins are indistinct, blending with adjacent edematous tissue. Note the ventricular compression and midline shift.

hemorrhage are prominent features. The mean survival time is only 11 months. Grades II and III are intermediate in both histologic features and survival time. Grading may also be applied to oligodendrogliomas and ependymomas, but with less well-defined clinical correlation.

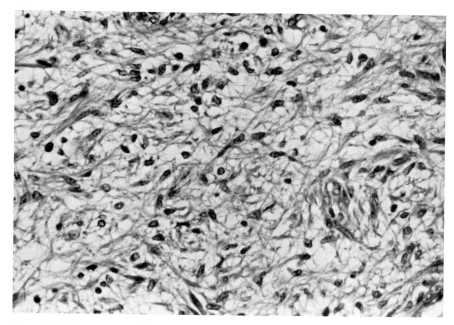

Figure 10.2. Astrocytoma, Grade I. Cells are relatively uniform and are readily identified as astrocytes. (Hematoxylin-phloxine-saffron (HPS), × 350).

Another widely accepted method of expressing the histologic appearance is based on a supposed resemblance of the tumor cells to the glia seen at various stages of differentiation in embryonic and fetal brain. In these classifications (there are many modifications), the least malignant tumors, composed predominantly of cells resembling mature glial elements, are called, simply, astrocytomas, oligodendrogliomas, or ependymomas. In the case of astrocytomas, adjectives such as fibrous, gemistocytic, piloid, or protoplasmic are often added. More malignant tumors are called astroblastomas, oligodendroglioblastomas, and ependymoblastomas; the most malignant tumors, corresponding roughly to Grades III and IV, are referred to as glioblastoma multiforme. Although at one time it was believed that the various tumors arose from undifferentiated precursor cells somehow retained in the brain from the intrauterine period, this view is now largely discredited. Experimental studies have provided considerable evidence that the neoplastic cells of gliomas are derived from previously normal glia, and that the morphologic appearance is an expression of the degree of malignancy rather than developmental origin.

Medulloblastomas are usually classified with the gliomas. They are

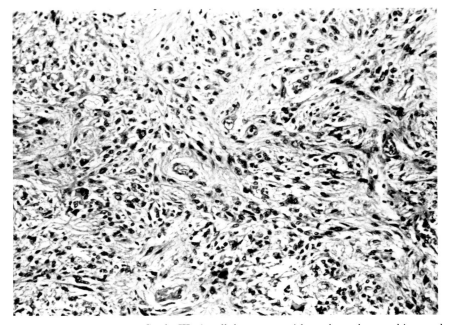

Figure 10.3. Astrocytoma, Grade III. A cellular tumor with nuclear pleomorphism and hyperchromasia, several giant cells, and areas of necrosis. (HPS), × 130.

relatively common tumors of children and young adults which probably arise from remnants of the external granular layer of the cerebellar cortex, the source of both neurons and glia in the developing cerebellum. The cells of the medulloblastoma are very small and lack distinctive features, although both neuroblastic and glial differentiation occurs to some degree. These tumors behave in two unusual ways when compared with other gliomas: they have a very great tendency to spread through cerebrospinal fluid pathways, and they are very responsive to radiotherapy.

Microgliomas are quite distinct in that they are not neuroectodermal in nature but are either closely related or identical to reticulum cell sarcoma. They are rare, infiltrate widely through the brain (Fig. 10.4), and are rapidly fatal within a few months of the first symptoms. There may be evidence of the lymphoma elsewhere in the body.

There are a number of less common glial or neuroectodermal tumors which will not be considered in this monograph.

MENINGIOMAS

The initial symptoms of meningiomas usually occur in middle-aged and elderly individuals, and the frequency is somewhat greater in fe-

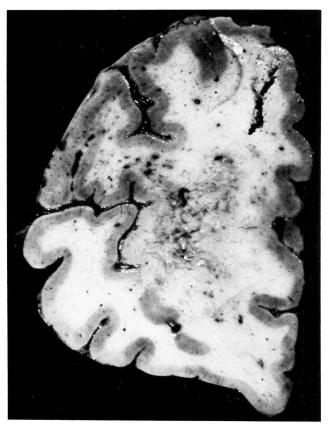

Figure 10.4. Infiltrating cerebral microglioma of frontal lobe with necrosis and hemorrhage. Patient first presented with a disturbance of behavior, 6 months before death.

males than in males. These tumors arise from the arachnoid lining cells and cells forming the arachnoid villi, and, rarely, the tela choroidea of the choroid plexuses.

Meningiomas are slow-growing, discrete tumors which compress, rather than invade, the adjacent brain (Fig. 10.5). However, they frequently invade adjacent bone and dura and may involve dural venous sinuses. The bony involvement may produce characteristic radiologic findings including hyperostosis or, more rarely, an osteolytic lesion. Histologically, the cells resemble those of arachnoid granulations (Fig. 10.6).

Most meningiomas can be removed surgically with success. Even when small bits of tumor are left adjacent to a venous sinus, recurrence

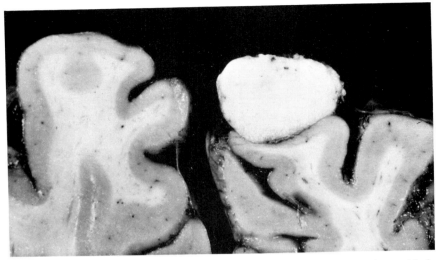

Figure 10.5. Small parasagittal meningioma found incidentally at autopsy in an elderly female. Note that the underlying gray matter is compressed but not invaded.

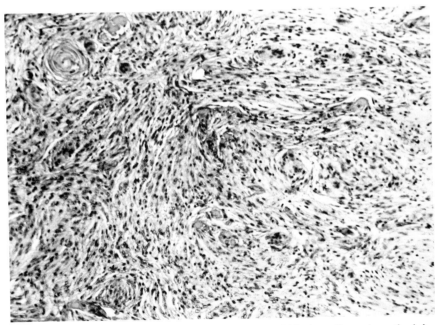

Figure 10.6. Meningioma. Interlacing fascicles of elongated bipolar cells, and, on the *left*, areas of plumper "epithelial" cells with more abundant cytoplasm. A meningothelial whorl composed of obsolete cells is at the *upper left*. (Hematoxylin-eosin, × 120)

usually requires many years and can again be resected. Remote metastases from malignant variants have been reported but are extremely uncommon. In a patient with evidence of an intracranial tumor, it is essential that meningiomas (or other resectable types of tumor) are differentiated, preferably by surgical biopsy, from the essentially untreatable gliomas and secondary tumors.

SCHWANNOMAS

Schwannomas (neurilemomas) are tumors of Schwann cells and occur anywhere along the course of cranial or peripheral nerves where the peripheral type of ensheathment is present. They are usually benign, encapsulated tumors attached to the nerve of origin. The malignant equivalent (neurogenic sarcoma) occurs occasionally.

The most frequent intracranial site is the acoustic nerve (Fig. 10.7), although the trigeminal and other nerves are occasionally involved. Intradural spinal nerve roots, particularly in the thoracic region, are also common locations.

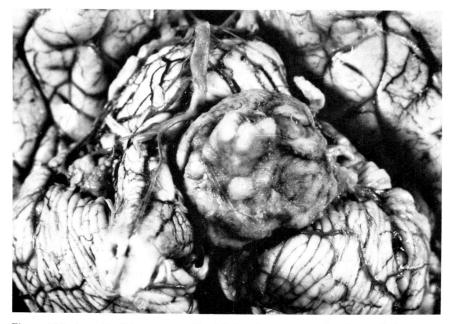

Figure 10.7. Acoustic Schwannoma. The lobulated tumor occupies the cerebellopontine angle, and has compressed and distorted the adjacent pons and medulla. The seventh and eighth cranial nerves were compressed on its upper surface, producing ipsilateral facial weakness and deafness.

MANIFESTATIONS OF TUMORS
General Effects

If a tumor grows slowly and infiltrates rather than destroys tissue, symptoms will evolve slowly and may be overlooked by the casual observer. Tumors produce symptoms and signs by two basic mechanisms:

1. The tumor mass and edema of surrounding tissues produce elevation of intracranial pressure leading to symptoms of intracranial hypertension, intracranial herniations, and finally compression of the brainstem. These general effects of raised intracranial pressure will be the same irrespective of the nature of the tumor, differing only in the rate of progression. The mechanisms and clinical effects of increased intracranial pressure are discussed in Chapter 3.

2. Focal disturbances are the result of compression, irritation, or destruction of adjacent tissue and lead to seizures or other symptoms of focal neurologic dysfunction. In addition to the general effects of raised intracranial pressure, symptoms characteristic of involvement of one or more areas of the central nervous system may appear and assist the clinician in localizing the lesion.

Seizures are the first symptom in about one-third of all cases of cerebral tumor. They may be generalized without localizing features, or they may reflect the area of the nervous system in which the tumor is situated and take the form of focal motor, sensory, or other types of seizures. Frequent or continuous seizures (status epilepticus) raise strongly the possibility of underlying neoplastic disease. In any patient suffering from epilepsy, a change in the nature of seizures or increasing resistance to anti-convulsant drug treatment suggests an underlying progressive lesion.

Disturbances in mental state may occur with tumors located above or below the tentorium but are more common with involvement of the cerebral hemispheres. Damage to the frontal lobes often leads to deterioration in social behavior, carelessness in personal appearance, and euphoria. The patient's mood may change, causing him to become irresponsible and unpredictable in his actions, or, on the other hand, dull and apathetic. If the lesion is in the leading hemisphere for speech, the patient may experience a defect in the inner formulation and expression of language (aphasia). Lesions involving the pre-central sulcus and the corticospinal tracts will lead to motor weakness on the opposite side of the body, most pronounced in the face and hand, with associated hyperreflexia and extensor plantar response (Babinski reflex). Stimulating the palm of the patient's hand may lead to reflex grasping.

Involvement of the parietal lobe can lead to complex symptoms. The parietal lobe is concerned with the integration of sensory information. Damage in this area leads to disturbances in cortical sensation over the opposite side of the body, including postural sensibility, tactile localization and discrimination, and sense of shape and form (astereognosis). Minor disturbances result in the patient's being unaware of one of two sensory stimuli applied simultaneously to both sides of the body (sensory inattention). Lesions in the left parietal lobe frequently produce aphasia and a disturbance in mathematical calculation and in naming body parts, whereas those in the right hemisphere may lead to an inability to dress in the absence of significant weakness (dressing apraxia) or denial of an obvious motor defect.

Lesions in the occipital lobe may produce seizures ushered in with a visual aura (warning) and the patient will show a defect in visual field testing if the optic radiations are involved. A patient with an homonymous hemianopia may not be aware of the defect.

Temporal lobe tumors will produce an upper quadrantic hemianopia if the lower fibers of the optic radiation are involved as they pass near the inferior horn of the lateral ventricle. A disturbance in understanding spoken language may appear if the posterior part of the temporal lobe in the dominant hemisphere is involved. The temporal lobe is also concerned with memory so that seizures arising from this region may be characterized by vivid recollection of past events.

Tumors located deep in the cerebral hemispheres and spreading bilaterally through the corpus callosum result in severe dementia, the basis for which may go unrecognized for some time.

Tumors deep in the substance of the hemispheres involve the internal capsule with motor, sensory, or visual symptoms resulting from damage to the major fiber pathways. Neoplastic growth in the basal ganglia rarely produces the extrapyramidal symptoms which develop in degenerative or infectious diseases of those regions.

Neoplasms in the region of the pineal body and third ventricle (Fig. 10.8) may produce internal hydrocephalus. On occasions there may be a disturbance in the patient's growth pattern or other endocrine dysfunction. Disturbed ocular function results when there is damage to the nearby superior colliculi and their connections.

No matter where a tumor may be located, the clinical picture is usually one of slow steady deterioration of neurologic function, occasionally punctuated with epileptiform attacks and often with the symptomatic background characteristic of rising intracranial pressure.

Clinical diagnosis and localization of a cerebral tumor may be aided by the findings of electroencephalography (Fig. 10.9). Brain scans using radioactive materials will reveal areas of abnormal vascular permeability

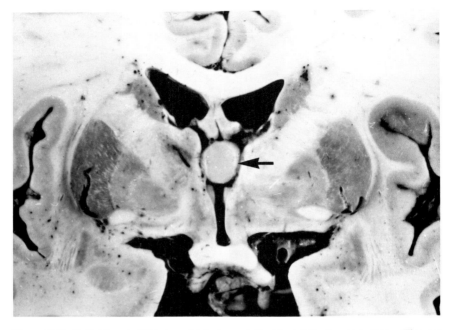

Figure 10.8. Colloid cyst of third ventricle (*arrow*). Incidental finding at autopsy. The cyst consists of a thin-walled fluid-filled sac, probably derived from the embryonic paraphysis, located at the level of the foramina of Monro. Larger cysts may produce intermittent or complete obstruction of the foramina with intracranial hypertension and hydrocephalus.

which occur in the vicinity of the tumors (Fig. 10.10) as well as in other lesions, for example infarcts, in which permeability is increased. Angiography (Fig. 10.11) and air encephalography will reveal space-occupying lesions as the result of the attendant displacements and distortions and intracranial structures.

Although any tumor may occur at almost any site and at any age, certain general groupings can be made on the basis of probability.

Tumors in Children

In children, tumors are particularly frequent in the posterior fossa near the fourth ventricle, and are most often medulloblastomas, ependymomas (Fig. 10.12), or low-grade astrocytomas. The early manifestations are frequently those of hydrocephalus due to obstruction of cerebrospinal fluid flow. This may lead to separation of cranial sutures and enlargement of the head.

If the tumor involves the midline of the cerebellum, the child will manifest ataxia of gait, and may have a tendency to fall backward. With

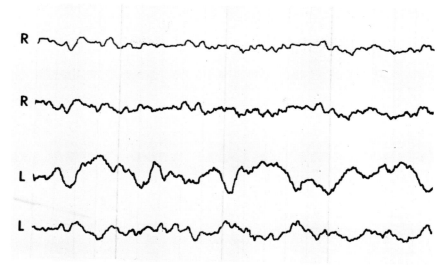

Figure 10.9. Electroencephalogram of a male, age 53, with a 1 year history of mild personality change, and dysphasia for 2 months. The two *upper* leads are from the right cerebral hemisphere, and the two *lower* ones from the left. Note the continuous slow wave abnormality from the left hemisphere, a characteristic electrical finding of an underlying destructive lesion. Biopsy showed an astrocytoma, Grade III.

involvement of the cerebellar hemispheres, examination reveals nystagmus, ipsilateral limb ataxia, and diminished resistance to passive movement (hypotonia). There may be a disturbance in head posture. Cranial nerves may be compressed on the side of the lesion.

Tumor growth in the brainstem leads to involvement of the cranial nerves and any of the ascending or descending tracts (Fig. 10.13). There may be involvement of ipsilateral cranial nerves with crossed motor or sensory signs on the opposite half of the body. Diplopia is a common first symptom. Cerebellar signs may appear as a result of damage to connecting pathways located in the brainstem.

These childhood tumors are occasionally responsive to therapy. Hydrocephalus can be temporarily relieved by shunting procedures. Medulloblastomas and some ependymomas are radiosensitive. The cerebellar astrocytomas are frequently well-localized cystic tumors which are resectable with good eventual return of function and, occasionally, permanent cure.

Tumors in Young Adults

In adults under the age of 50, the majority of tumors are gliomas of the cerebral hemispheres, and of these, half or more are the highly malig-

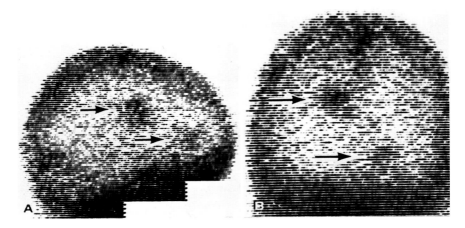

Figure 10.10. A and *B:* brain scan of a female, age 20, with right hemiplegia and slurring of speech of 1 month duration. Previous history of carcinoma of the breast. Scan reveals two focal areas of increased permeability to the marker (Technetium ^{99}M) in the frontal lobes bilaterally (*arrows*).

nant glioblastoma multiforme. Because of the wide range of malignancy, however, a histologic diagnosis is usually undertaken for prognostic purposes and to exclude less common but potentially treatable neoplasms.

Tumors in the Elderly

Metastatic tumors, particularly from carcinoma of the lung, breast, thyroid, gastrointestinal tract, and prostate are common in this age group (Figs. 10.14, 10.15). Investigative and therapeutic problems arise when, as occasionally happens, the cerebral metastasis is manifest at a stage when a primary lesion cannot yet be identified.

Among the primary intracranial tumors, meningiomas are probably the most frequent; gliomas and other types occasionally occur.

Tumors at the Base of the Brain

Cranipharyngiomas are squamous epithelial tumors derived from Rathke's pouch remnants in the vicinity of the sella turcica, usually occurring in children and young adults. These, and pituitary adenomas, meningiomas, and a variety of less common tumors occurring in this vicinity, commonly produce syndromes in which evidences of endocrine and hypothalamic dysfunction are combined with neurologic manifestations of compression or invasion of optic nerves and chiasm, diencephalic structures, and the third, fourth, and sixth cranial nerves.

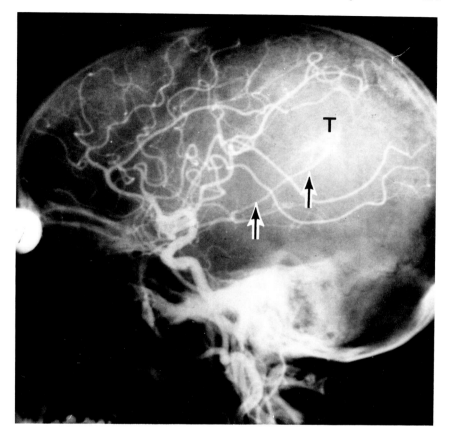

Figure 10.11. Cerebral angiogram of a male, age 55, with a history of occasional focal left-sided motor seizures for 5 years and recent complaint of morning headache. Examination showed mild papilledema. Angiogram reveals separation and displacement of the posterior cortical branches of the right middle cerebral artery. The tumor (*T*), which was a meningioma, receives its blood supply from an enlarged posterior branch of the middle meningeal artery (*arrows*).

Tumors of the Spinal Cord

Spinal cord tumors may be divided, according to their location, into extradural or intradural growths with the latter further divided into those arising within the cord (intramedullary) or outside of the cord (extramedullary). Schwannomas, menigiomas, and gliomas all occur with about equal frequency, with 10 percent being a miscellaneous group of chordomas and other uncommon tumors. The majority of tumors occur in the thoracic region and usually appear in patients be-

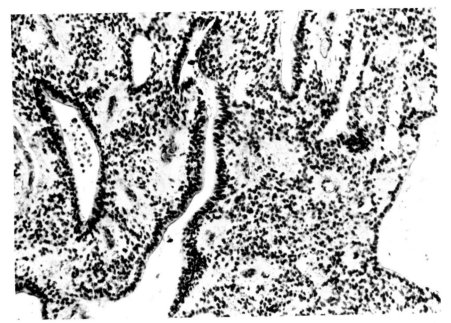

Figure 10.12. Ependymoma. Female, age 11. The tumor filled the lower portion of the fourth ventricle and had produced hydrocephalus and cerebellar signs. The tumor cells form cavities and clefts lined by ependyma-like epithelium, between which is a random array of neoplastic glial cells, with some tendency to perivascular rosette formation. (Phosphotungstic acid-hematoxylin, × 130)

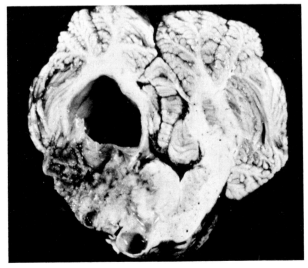

Figure 10.13. Astrocytoma of pons and cerebellum. Infant, age 1 year; progressive hemiplegia and multiple cranial nerve palsies. The tumor has infiltrated and destroyed much of the pons, middle cerebellar peduncle on the *left*, and adjacent cerebellar hemisphere; in the latter region it has led to formation of a large cyst. The tumor exhibits necrosis and hemorrhage.

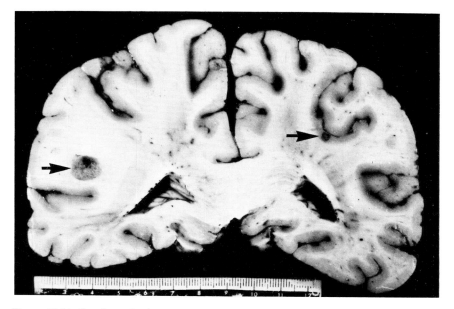

Figure 10.14. Small cerebral metastases from oat-cell carcinoma of lung (*arrows*). Note the very marked edema of the adjacent white matter on the *left;* the displacement of midline structures is largely the result of edema rather than tumor mass. The clinical manifestations were similarly out of proportion to the rather minimal tissue destruction.

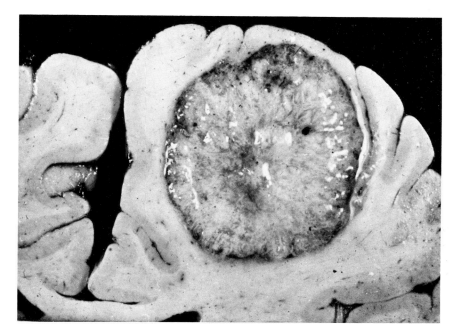

Figure 10.15. Large cerebral metastasis from carcinoma of colon. The lesion is sharply demarcated from the surrounding cerebral tissue.

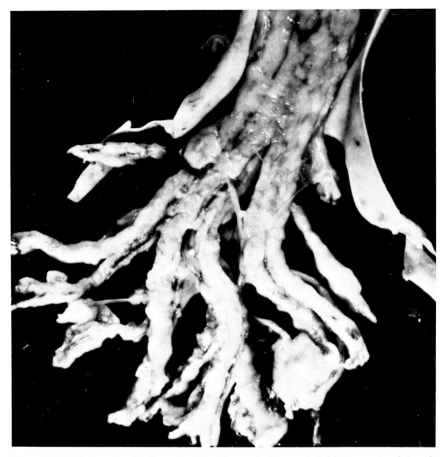

Figure 10.16. Subarachnoid dissemination of a cerebellar medulloblastoma, involving the nerve roots of the cauda equina.

tween the ages of 20 and 60 years. Since Schwannomas and meningiomas are usually curable, early diagnosis is essential.

Secondary carcinoma of the vertebral column may produce spinal cord compression as a result of invasion of the extradural space or collapse of the vertebrae. The prostate and breast are commonly the primary sites. Lymphomas, notably lymphosarcoma and Hodgkin's disease, may involve either the extradural or intradural structures.

The symptoms of spinal cord damage will depend upon the speed of development, location, and, to a lesser degree, the nature of the tumor. The spinal cord appears able to compensate for lengthy periods of time, followed by rapid deterioration. In any patient with the clinical picture

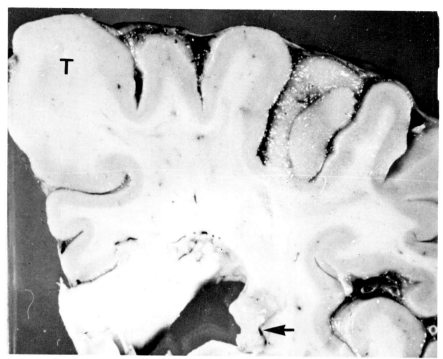

Figure 10.17. Tuberous sclerosis. Male, age 14. History of mental retardation and seizures from age 2. Large cortical hamartoma (the tuber) (*T*) which was composed of disorganized glial and neural cells, often abnormal in configuration. Note absence of normal cortical appearance in the region. A subependymal glial hamartoma protrudes into the lateral ventricle (*arrow*). The periventricular hamartomas occasionally give origin to astrocytomas.

of a rapidly progressive spinal cord lesion, immediate investigation is mandatory since compression by either a neoplasm or intervertebral disc is potentially treatable before irreversible cord damage occurs.

Sensory disturbance and later weakness at and below the level of the lesion are cardinal features of spinal cord involvement. If nerve roots are compressed, there will be pain at the level of the lesion and there may be tenderness to pressure applied to the vertebral column. The sensory disturbance usually does not affect all forms of sensation to the same degree, but a level can usually be found above which all forms of sensation are normal. Pyramidal tract damage causes weakness, increased resistance to passive movement (spasticity), and augmentation of the deep tendon reflexes. The distribution of weakness and pattern of reflex abnormalities will be of localizing value to the clinician familiar with the segmental innervation of muscles.

Impairment of sphincter control develops as a late and sometimes ominous complication.

The spinal cord ends at the lower border of the first lumbar vertebra below which lesions will involve the roots of the cauda equina, causing nerve root pain, flaccid paraplegia, absent reflexes, and sensory loss with bladder involvement (Fig. 10.16).

ETIOLOGY OF BRAIN TUMORS

The vast majority of intracranial tumors occur apparently spontaneously without known predisposing environmental or genetic factors.

There are, however, a number of hereditary syndromes in which tumors of the nervous system occur with high frequency (Fig. 10.17). Some of these are the following:

Name	*Transmission*	*Principal features*	*Tumors*
Multiple neurofibromatosis (Von Recklinghausen's disease)	Dominant	Multiple neurofibromas of skin and viscera; patches of cutaneous pigmentation	Neurilemomas; neurogenic sarcomas; meningiomas; optic nerve gliomas
Tuberous sclerosis (Bourneville's disease)	Dominant	Multiple hamartomas of brain, heart, kidney, lung, skin, and elsewhere	Gliomas, usually paraventricular
Cerebelloretinal angiomatosis (Lindau-Von Hippel syndrome)	Dominant	Angiomas of retina, skin, and elsewhere; renal and pancreatic cysts and adenomas; occasionally renal carcinomas	Cerebellar and spinal hemangioblastomas
Neurocutaneous melanosis	Dominant	Hyperpigmentation of face, eye, and meninges	Malignant melanomas of meninges

In experimental animals, brain tumors are readily induced by a number of oncogenic viruses, particularly polyoma, SV40, and Rous sarcoma viruses. Most of these tumors are sarcomas, but a few neuroectodermal tumors are produced as well. As in many other systems, the virus is difficult or impossible to recover from the established tumors.

A number of chemical carcinogens given to animals orally, systemically, or by implantation produce gliomas or sarcomas. Pellets of methylcholanthrene implanted in the brain are highly carcinogenic, giving rise to a wide range of gliomas often containing a mixture of several histologic cell types.

Recently, the observation of virus-like particles in chemically-induced gliomas has attracted considerable attention in regard to possible interaction between the two agents, but this awaits further study.

REFERENCES

HARKIN, J. C., AND REED, R. J. Tumors of the Peripheral Nervous System. Armed Forces Institute of Pathology, Second Series, Fascicle 3, Washington, 1969.

KERNOHAN, J. W., AND SAYRE, G. P. Tumors of the Central Nervous System. Armed Forces Institute of Pathology, Fascicle 35, Washington, 1952.

KERNOHAN, J. W., AND UIHLEIN, A. Sarcomas of the Brain. Charles C Thomas, Publisher, Inc., Springfield, Ill., 1962.

RUSSELL, D. S., AND RUBINSTEIN, L. J. Pathology of Tumors of the Nervous System. Edward Arnold, Ltd., London, 1971.

VICK, N. A., BIGNER, D. D., AND KVEDAR, J. P. The fine structure of canine gliomas and intracranial sarcomas induced by the Schmidt-Ruppin strain of the Rous sarcoma virus. J. Neuropath. Exp. Neurol. 30:354, 1971.

ZIMMERMAN, H. M., NETSKY, M. G., AND DAVIDOFF, L. M. Atlas of Tumors of the Nervous System. Lea & Febiger, Philadelphia, 1956.

ZÜLCH, K. J. Brain Tumors. Their Biology and Pathology. Springer, New York, 1965.

INDEX

Arnold-Chiari, 54
hydrocephalus due to, 52
virus-induced, 131
Malnutrition, effects on brain, 69
Measles
associated with para-infectious encephalitis, 113
in multiple sclerosis, 106
subacute sclerosing panencephalitis, 136
Medulloblastomas, 183–184, 190, 191
Melanosis, neurocutaneous, 198
Meninges
fibrosis, 52, 55, 103
hemorrhage
extradural, 147–148
subarachnoid, 98, 102
subdural, 149–152
infections
abscess, epidural and subdural, 122–123
leptomeningitis, 123–125
neoplasms
infiltration by, 122
meningioma, 184–187, 192, 193
Meningiomas, 184–187, 192, 193
Meningitis, *see* Leptomeningitis
Mental deficiency, 63
Microglia, 28–30, 31, 33
neuronophagia, 29
origin, 28
reactions, 29
rod cells, 29
Microgliomas, 184, 185
Microinfarction, cerebral, 89–90
Midbrain
changes in Parkinson's disease, 169–170
compression by tentorial herniation, 40–45
concussion, 144–155
Motor neuron
in motor neuron disease, 174–177
lower, 5, 6
upper, 5
Multiple sclerosis, 105–113
clinical findings, 109–112
etiology, 106, 107
lipid breakdown in, 33, 34
mild forms, 113
myelin sheaths in, 31, 107
pathologic features, 107, 108
Mumps virus, causing aqueduct stenosis, 131
Mycotic infections, 128–130
Myelin sheaths, 30–34
breakdown, 31–32

destruction, mechanisms of, 30, 31
phagocytosis, 32
regeneration, 32–34

Necrosis
brainstem, due to compression, 40, 42–46
in infarction, 87–89
in viral infections, 132, 133
of neurons, 16
pseudolaminar, 68, 69
Negri bodies, 18
Neoplasms, extracranial
metastases to central nervous system, 192, 195
remote effects upon nervous system, 137–139
Neoplasms, intracranial, 180–199
classification, 180–181
experimental production, 198–199
general manifestations, 188–192
hemorrhage into, 94
herniations produced by, 39, 40
increased intracranial pressure, 37
inheritance, 198
meningeal infiltration, 122
Neoplasms, intraspinal, 193–198
Neurilemomas, 187
Neurocutaneous melanosis, 198
Neurofibrillary degeneration, 18, 161–162
Neurofibromatosis, multiple, 198
Neuromyelitis optica, 112
Neuronophagia, 29, 33
Neurons, reactions in disease, 16–23
artifacts, 16
atrophy, 17
axonal reaction, 22
central chromatolysis, 22, 23
depletion, 16
inclusions, 17
necrosis, 16
neurofibrillary degeneration, 18
swelling, 16
Neuropathy
acute infectious, 115–117
carcinomatous, 138
experimentally induced, 118
nutritional, 70
peroneal muscular atrophy, 178
segmental, 34
uremic, 76
Neuropil, 15

Oligodendroglia, 26, 27
conversion, 27